This book

informs persons who have sustained or risk a heart attack as a result of coronary artery disease how it is possible to help them and how they may help themselves.

In this new volume of the *Medical Adviser Series* two experienced cardiologists, who have been involved for many years in research of the causes and consequences of this disease, give a comprehensive description of heart attack and its effects. They answer questions which are brought up daily by those who are affected by heart attack and coronary disease in general.

Yet another purpose of this book is to make patients specialists of their particular chronic disease with the cooperation of their physician. The book is meant to become a reliable adviser on the way to a 'second life', one which may be consulted at any time by patients and their families.

Carola Halhuber, M.D.

Born in 1936 in Baden-Baden, Dr. Halhuber received her medical education at the Universities of Freiburg, Vienna, Berlin and Munster.

She was head of the Clinic of Cardio-vascular Disease in Baden-Baden and of the private Hospital "Lauterbacher Muehle" for coronary patients at Osterseen in Bavaria from 1964 to 1974. Since 1974 she has worked in the intensive care unit of the County Hospital in Munich-Pasing.

She is a trustee member of the German society concerned with the dangers of addiction, speaker for a group of specialists on smoking, and head of an outpatient coronary group.

Max J. Halhuber, M.D., Professor of Medicine

Born in 1916 in Innsbruck, Dr. Haluber studied medicine in Innsbruck, Vienna, Freiburg, Paris, and Boston.

He was chief resident of the University Hospital in Innsbruck until 1967. Since 1968 he has been the medical director of the Hoehenried Hospital for Cardio-vascular Disease.

He is professor of medicine at the University of Innsbruck and the Technical University of Munich.

Carola Halhuber, M.D.
Prof. Max J. Halhuber, M.D.

Speaking of:

Heart
Attacks

**Early recognition, Rehabilitation,
Prevention of Recurrence**

Comprehensive Guide for Coronary Patients

with a preface by Robert M. Kohn, M.D.

Translation: Françoise Heyden

Consolidated Book Publishers

NEW YORK • CHICAGO

Library of Congress Catalog Card Number: 78-72876
ISBN: 0-8326-2232-X

Originally published in German under the title *Sprechs-
tunde: Herzinfarkt,* copyright © 1978 by Gräfe und
Unzer Verlag, München.

Contents

Preface

In Germany the patient with a heart attack is referred to a special center for cardiac rehabilitation after his hospitalization for acute care. One such center in Bavaria is run by Dr. Max Halhuber who shares his experience and knowledge with us in this book, written for the patient and his family.

In the United States we have superb facilities for care during the acute phase of the heart attack. However, we neglect the important rehabilitation and reconditioning process and put up with the high cost, both socially and economically, of prolonged disability and premature retirement.

A statement was made to me by one of the officials of a Blue Shield plan when challenged over the Blue Plan's policy of not paying for a rehabilitation program. He stated, "The Blue Plans are in business to insure against acute illness. We are not in the business of prevention nor in the business of rehabilitation, much as we applaud their aims." If the individual is fortunate enough to have major medical coverage, rehabilitation programs may be covered.

It is unfortunate in these days of pressures for cost containment in medical care that we neglect rehabilitation and secondary prevention. As a matter of fact, even primary prevention programs suffer.

It has been estimated that in the United States coronary disease strikes 2½ million individuals, and that one in five men can expect to have a heart attack before age 60. While institutional rehabilitation will probably never come to this country, and, indeed, is probably not needed, we must find a higher priority for prevention and rehabilitation programs.

Dr. Halhuber has a lot to tell us about coronary artery disease and heart attacks, and this book offers a large amount of medical information in terms understandable by patients and their family.

Robert M. Kohn, M.D.
Clinical Professor of Medicine
State University of New York at
* Buffalo*

Director, Buffalo Cardiac Work
* Evaluation Unit*
Editor, Cardiac Rehabilitation
Quarterly

Why This Book Is Important to Us

All questions with which we are concerned in this book were raised by our patients. Our primary reason for writing this book is that most of the answers to these questions were to be found only in medical journals not easily accessible to the layman.

Cooperation between physician and patient

The second reason is that we consider the cooperation of the patient with his doctor to be very important. Experience with treating patients over the years has convinced us that the treatment is always more successful if there is cooperation between the well-informed patient and his physician. Information gained in this manner is a crucial prerequisite in motivating the patient to comply with long-term medication and to undergo the often necessary changes in life-style.

We thus advocate the well-informed patient who becomes a specialist concerning his particular chronic disease. For this reason, everything which is discussed in this volume of the *Medical Adviser Series* is described in a manner comprehensible to the medical layman.

It is unavoidable that such a description is oversimplified. Perhaps we could be criticized because oversimplification can lead to incorrect information, but we must insist that such a description is justified as long as it helps the patient to better understand his particular chronic disease.

In our opinion, a mature patient is not only well-informed, but also one who has the basic right to make his own decisions, even if these are not in accordance with our medical advice.

We have taken it upon ourselves to write a reliable guide for the coronary patient and his family in the hope that we may alleviate some of the constantly pressing problems. In this respect our experience over the years in the comprehensive long-term treatment and rehabilitation of coronary patients prior to, as well as after the heart attack, has proven to be valuable. We have gained insight in treatment methods in our experience with thousands of patients in general hospitals, rehabilitation centers, as well as in private clinics and through discussions with our colleagues.

For whom is this book written?

What kind of reading audience did we have in mind while writing this volume of the *Medical Adviser Series?* Who would gain most from reading our book? The book is intended above all for those who have sustained a heart attack, but do not understand why it occurred and wonder what to expect next. Secondly, the book is meant for those who suspect that they are developing coronary problems and would like to take measures to prevent a heart attack before it is too late. Thirdly, we aim our book at the relatives of coronary patients, because we are well aware of the important role the sympathy and encouragement of friends can play in the convalescence of the patient. Frequently the family of the coronary patient hinders rehabilitation because fear and misunderstanding sometimes result from the physician's warnings and advice.

Prerequisites for a normal life

The goal of all such precautionary measures is longevity combined with the best possible quality of life. This goal may be achieved by the coronary patient as by the diabetic through discipline and adoption of the appropriate life-style. The patient may then return to a normal life which may in fact be happier and more satisfactory than it was prior to the heart attack.

The fact that we frequently meet former coronary patients on ski or mountain climbing trips has shown us that sports may play an important role in the happiness of former patients whose activities should not be restricted by overemphasis of caution. (This introductory chapter was originally entitled "On Glacier Tours with Coronary Patients".) We have evidence, and can confirm with case histories, that patients are able to tolerate physical activity at 6,500 feet—if the guidelines prescribed in this book are followed. However, this one aspect is perhaps too specific for the scope of this book.

We hope to advance the opinion that it is possible, more often than generally assumed, for coronary patients to resume the normal lives characteristic of their particular age.

It is not by mere accident that we have borrowed the term *rehabilitation* from pedagogy to emphasize the educational aspect, because rehabilitation must include self-growth and respect for others.

What we mean by this generalized, almost philosophical, affirmation will be clarified by a careful reading of our book.

An unusual writing process

In many respects the writing of this book was unusual. The table of contents was discussed with coronary patients in the private clinic "Lauterbacher Muhle". The patients specified which pertinent information needed to be included, which chapters were of particular interest to them, and what kind of questions were of great importance. Moreover, we revised each chapter with the help of the editor in order to make certain that the text would be easily understood by laymen without, however, sacrificing medical accuracy. At this point we would therefore like to thank the publishers as well as Mrs. Schimmelpfennig-Funke and Mr. Scherz for their patience, understanding, and cooperation, Françoise Heyden for the good translation, and Robert M. Kohn for supervising the American edition of this book.

In closing the authors would like to mention that this book means more to them than many of their other writings.

Carola and Max J. Halhuber

1. What Is a Heart Attack and Why Does It Occur?

A heart attack is a sudden, local blockage of the blood circulation in the coronary artery. As a result, there is such a great lack of oxygen in the cells of the heart muscle that they die. In 95% of such cases, changes in the structure of the coronary arteries are the cause of the acute imbalance between the demand for oxygen in the heart and the blood supply of oxygen. (This condition is sometimes mistakenly referred to as hardening of the arteries, implying calcification of the arterial wall, even though calcium deposits are rarely the major cause and should be considered secondary.)

Changes in the structure of the coronaries

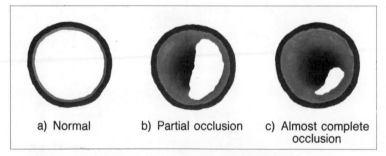

a) Normal   b) Partial occlusion   c) Almost complete occlusion

The three cross-sections of a coronary vessel show:
a) a normal opening without changes in the vessel walls
b) a partial occlusion due to thickening of the vessel wall at this point
c) a further stage in the development of coronary heart disease

What is the function of these coronary vessels which originate at the base of the aorta and form a net-work throughout the heart muscle? The heart muscle which is the size of a fist and which pumps blood into the vessels by contraction (systole) must be furnished with blood through special arteries just like every organ of the body. Heart attacks develop most frequently as a result of the occlusion of a coronary artery, the function of which is to supply a certain area of the heart muscle with oxygen.

Thickening of vessels and blood clots

What causes such an occlusion? It is most often the result of thickening of the arterial wall and of blood clotting. However, blood clots usually develop only after a slowing down of the blood

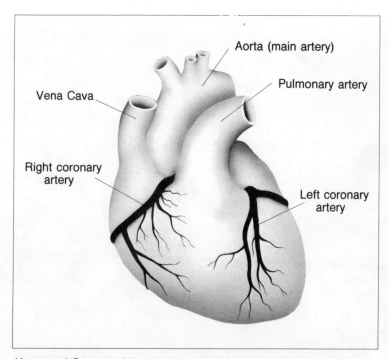

Heart and Coronary Vessels. The vessels which nourish the heart originate at the base of the aorta. While the right coronary vessel supplies the back wall, the left coronary artery nourishes the anterior and side wall of the heart.

flow in the vessels. If the blood supply to any area of the myocardium (heart muscle) is blocked, then the affected area may die. Should an occlusion occur in a larger branch, then a larger area of the myocardium will die. On the other hand, the smaller the blocked branch is, the less severe the heart attack. Such minor heart attacks are, of course, much easier to overcome than major attacks. But even extensive muscle damage from severe heart attacks may heal well. In other words, heart attacks are not to be judged on an equal basis.

A heart attack rarely occurs completely unexpectedly or suddenly without any warning. Such warning signs may take the

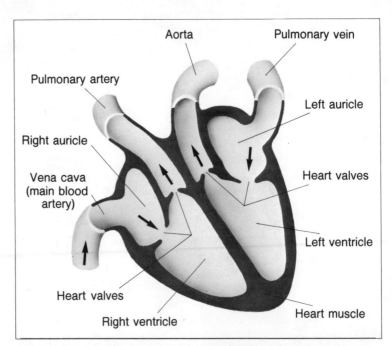

Heart cut length-wise to show direction of blood flow. Oxygen depleted blood returns to the heart via the vena cava and the right auricle. It passes through the three-pointed cardiac valve (tricuspid) into the right ventricle. The right ventricle pumps the blood into the pulmonary artery and its branches. Thus the blood is oxygenated again and passes through the pulmonary veins into the left auricle. The blood then flows through the two pointed cardiac valve (mitral) into the left ventricle. The left ventricle pumps the blood into the aorta and the branches, i.e. major arteries. Between both the right ventricle and pulmonary artery as well as between the left ventricle and aorta are the semilunar valves.

14

form of chest pains, that is, symptoms of angina pectoris (this
chest tightness can be called *stenocardia*) which increase in
frequency and intensity in the time period prior to the actual heart
attack. An acute coronary occlusion is often preceeded by a long
chronic stage of coronary heart disease (CHD) resulting in
changes in the vessel walls which impede the blood flow.

The thickening and subsequent narrowing of the blood vessel
walls is caused by various developments such as cholesterol
deposits and inflammatory reactions. In this manner the blood
supply to a particular area of the heart muscle is impaired, and
this blockage eventually leads to the occlusion of a coronary vessel
and the heart attack. (We are still not certain whether the
formation of a blood clot comes prior to or as a consequence of
the vessel occlusion. In any case, the prevention and treatment of
blood clots is of great importance.)

Causes for angina pectoris and heart attacks may be found in
the imbalance between oxygen demand and actual oxygen supply
by the blood vessels. Such a disproportion is evident to a smaller
degree in angina pectoris and to a larger degree in the case of

*Impaired
circulation*
heart attack. Impaired blood circulation may result not only when
the blood vessels do not supply sufficient oxygen, but also when
the heart muscle suddenly demands more oxygen (that is,
oxygenated blood). Such an increased demand may be the result
of physical exertion or emotional stress, as for example in a
frightening situation. In this case, the adrenal glands secrete a
hormone which is carried by the blood stream to the cells of the
heart muscle where it causes an increase in the oxygen demand of
the myocardial cells. This increased demand may in turn be one of
the reasons for the occurrence of angina pectoris and heart attack
in acute emotional stress. Moreover, it is suspected that cigarette
smoking can lead to the same consequences.

Since the causes of impaired circulation and increased oxygen
demand are to be found not simply in the thickening of blood
vessels, but instead in the interplay of the heart muscle and the

*Ischemic
heart disease*
coronary arteries, the term 'ischemic heart disease' (ischemic
means bloodless) is frequently substituted for 'coronary disease' in
current medical terminology. This differentiation is practical and is
psychologically significant because in prevention, as in treatment
of heart attacks, we must keep in mind all relevant factors.
Measures (such as physical exercise and emotional relaxation)
which may help to improve the total blood circulation thus

15

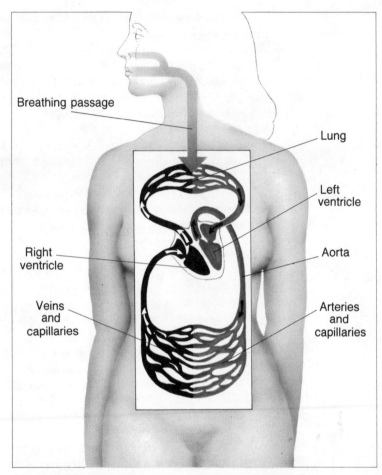

Breathing passage

Lung

Left ventricle

Right ventricle

Aorta

Veins and capillaries

Arteries and capillaries

The Heart and Blood Circulation. The heart consists of two independent ventricles and auricles. The right ventricle supplies blood to the circulation of the lung where it is enriched with oxygen. The left ventricle must pump the blood into the general circulation, the arteries and capillaries of which supply the body with blood and are simplified in this diagram.

economize the oxygen demand and supply of the heart muscle. In other words, the dangers of acutely impaired circulation can be avoided in this manner.

An analogy may be drawn between the distribution of coronary vessels in the myocardium and the branches of a tree. If a large branch of a tree is damaged, then the leaves which grow on this branch fall off. However, this comparison is incomplete because it does not account for the collateral blood vessels of the heart muscle. Although these collaterals do not function continually, they may be effectively enlarged by increased oxygen demand or physical exercise and may then aid in the prevention of a heart attack.

However, these collaterals which are also called anastomoses resemble a network of pathways more than branches of a tree. An analogy to a network of pathways is helpful in explaining how an acute blockage may suddenly develop as a result of a traffic jam or road repairs. (These may be comparable to the scar tissue repairs following the damage of a heart attack.) Such roadway blockages may be avoided by using detour roads, or, in this case, the collaterals. In fact, it has been shown that in man collaterals may not only be effectively used, but that previously unused collaterals then begin to function. The development of additional collaterals surrounding the area where there is scar tissue from a heart attack probably improves circulation and also leads to a diminishing or even the disappearance of the scar itself.

Economizing the general circulation

Two factors are important in preventing (primary prevention) and halting the progression of coronary disease. First, it is important to prevent changes in the blood vessel walls (i.e. arteriosclerosis not only in the coronary vessels, but in all organs.) Secondly, the unburdening of the myocardial work load by decreased oxygen demand is of equal importance. It is possible to attain these goals by means of medication as well as physical exercise.

The exact causes of arteriosclerosis have not been completely determined.

Nevertheless, it is certain that there is no single cause, but that there are instead a number of interacting factors in an unhealthy life-style which cause heart attack. These are referred to as the risk factors in coronary heart disease.

2. Risk Factors

Life-Style and Habits Which May Lead to a Heart Attack

Discovering and reducing risk factors

The term *risk factor** refers to certain living habits which cause disease or which are observed more frequently among coronary patients than among healthy persons. Although a specific cause and effect pattern may not be discernible in each individual case, it is nonetheless worthwhile to compile a risk profile in order that every person may determine and subsequently reduce his personal risk factors. Since the risk factors discussed in this chapter are of varying importance to the particular individual, the order of the risk factors is necessarily arbitrary.

The reader may ask, 'why'? It is known that fat metabolism plays an important role in the development of a heart attack, in fact a more significant role than high blood pressure. (In the case of stroke, on the contrary, high blood pressure is the primary risk factor.) But it is also known that many young people smoke and that cigarette smoking may entail grave consequences, particularly for the heavy smokers under the age of 40. Moreover, the contraceptive pill plays a decisive role for those women who are already in risk for other reasons, e.g. smoking and hypertension.

Risk Factor: Elevated Blood Fat Levels

Blood lipids (fats) provide energy and serve as building blocks for

---

* The term *risk factor* is employed in epidemiology which is the science of the distribution of disease in different populations.

18

the organism. The body not only composes its own fats, but also gets lipids directly from the food intake. The lipids are then transported to the various organs and tissues via the blood stream and are either burned or stored if there is no immediate use for them. Apparently the lipids invade the walls of blood vessels and thus lead to the development of arteriosclerosis. We add the word 'apparently' because the exact nature of the link between lipids and coronary arteriosclerosis has not been completely clarified. Animal experiments have proved conclusively that an increase in blood lipid levels leads to hardening of the arteries. In this process two kinds of lipids play an important role, cholesterol and triglycerides (neutral fats). For the most part cholesterol also depends on the various types of fat in our nutrition and the amount of cholesterol present in certain foods. (The highest level of cholesterol is found in egg yolks and butter, as well as in meats from inner organs such as brain and liver.) Moreover, the body can convert carbohydrates such as sugar, flour, and bread into fat (triglycerides). This conversion occurs in the liver as well as in adipose fat tissue. An elevated lipid level is the consequence of meals too high in fat and carbohydrate content. Since the blood fat level usually cannot normalize itself in the time period between meals, it remains elevated. It should also be mentioned that abnormal fat metabolism, also referred to as hyperlipidemia, is found in other diseases such as diabetes and abnormal liver, kidney and thyroid functioning. Clearly elevated lipid levels (cholesterol values above 260mg% and triglyceride values higher than 200mg%) are found in about 25% of all American adults. Do you also belong to the group with this risk factor?

Elevated cholesterol levels

Normal and elevated levels

Average Values for 40 Year Old Man	
Cholesterol Levels in the Blood	
normal:	less than 220mg%
borderline:	220 to 260mg%
elevated:	higher than 260mg%
Triglyceride Levels in the Blood	
normal:	less than 150mg%
borderline:	150 to 200mg%
elevated:	higher than 200mg%

Risk Factor: Low Levels of HDL—High levels of LDL—Cholesterol

Research over the past ten years has presented us with a much clearer insight into the problems involved with blood fats. It is now established that the total cholesterol level as measured in most laboratories correlates very well with a substance which is called "low density lipoprotein". What does the term 'low density lipoprotein' mean? First, it is important to realize that blood fats or lipids cannot float freely in the blood circulation; the lipids are bound to protein; therefore, they are termed lipo-proteins. With a special instrument, it is possible to measure these lipoproteins in their degree of density. Everyone has high density lipoproteins (abbreviated HDL) and low density lipoproteins (abbreviated LDL). Interestingly, HDL contains almost 50% protein and less than a quarter cholesterol, while LDL contains close to 50% cholesterol and less than a quarter of protein. From long-term observations it became quite clear that HDL levels, the higher they are, the more protective they seem to be from atheroscleortic heart disease. This is not surprising if one looks at all the factors, presently known to increase HDL levels (Table 1). The only disturbing observation is that pesticides, too, and estrogen therapy after menopause may increase HDL levels (and we are not sure at this time whether this is cause for concern). On the other hand, elevated LDL levels are found in individuals who are, from many aspects, at higher risk—but who could do something about most of the factors listed in the second table.

As the HDL table indicates, only race and sex obviously cannot be influenced, but all the things we ought to do are listed on the left side: preference of vegetable oils and margarine over butter and other animal fats, regular exercise, abstaining from smoking, using alcohol in moderation, keeping the weight normal, remaining at normal cholesterol, triglyceride and blood sugar levels. For the first time in the past 30 years of research in risk factors, a unifying concept has emerged which gives us the assurance that it is worthwhile to intervene if we have one or several risk factors. At the same time, the multifactorial aspect of this disease becomes so obvious that it would be foolish to expect any major impact on the primary or secondary prevention of

20

coronary heart disease if one would attempt to influence only one single risk factor.

The LDL table contains the gravest of all risk factors, hypercholesterolemia of the familial type, previously termed primary or essential or familial hypercholesterolemia, because it is running in families and has frequently wiped out entire generations even in adolescence. The survivors have carried the abnormal gene on to the next generation before succumbing to a heart attack usually in their thirties or forties. But the LDL levels are also elevated among smokers, inactive persons on a diet high in animal fat and more often seen in men than in women. Recently it was demonstrated that quitting smoking, taking up regular physical exercise and consuming a diet rich in vegetable oil, fish and skim milk products can definitely lower these LDL levels, thus contributing to a decrease in the overall risk for ischemic heart disease.

Table 1

HDL high increased	HDL low reduced
black race	white race
females	males
vegetables fats, oils	high animal fat diet
physical activity	physical inactivity
non- or ex-smoker	smoker
moderate alcohol intake	no alcohol intake
normal weight	obesity
normal cholesterol levels	hypercholesterolemia
low triglyceride levels	high triglyceride levels
normal glucose levels	diabetes mellitus
non-coronary persons	chd-patients
children, healthy parents	children of chd-patients
pesticides estrogens	

21

Table 2

LDL high increased	LDL low reduced
white race	black race
males	females
physical inactivity	physical activity
smoker	non- or ex-smoker
no alcohol intake	moderate alcohol intake
hypercholesterolemia	normal cholesterol concentration
high animal fat diet	polyunsaturated fatty acids
chd patients	non-coronary persons
impaired longevity	longevity

(This section on HDL-LDL, including the tables was kindly provided by S. Heyden, M.D., Ph.D., Professor of Community and Family Medicine at Duke University Medical Center, Durham, N.C.)

Risk Factor: Diabetes

The Framingham Study confirms the well-known fact that every second diabetic suffers from coronary disease. This finding emphasizes the danger of coronary disease to an undiagnosed or untreated diabetic. Examinations of diabetics show that arterial vascular disease is twice as frequent among them as compared to healthy persons. Dangers are greater for diabetic women than for men because of complications.

Diabetics are at risk

The Framingham Study also revealed that the average blood pressure values are higher among diabetic men, and even higher among diabetic women, than among the non-diabetic population. It follows that diabetics are especially at risk.

The most important goal of treatment of diabetic adults is the normalization of weight because diabetics frequently do not need medication if they maintain their normal weight and a proper diet.

Evaluation of blood glucose and urinary sugar
The diabetic and his physician must rely on repeated blood and urinary sugar tests for long-term treatment. The patient can learn

22

to perform these simple tests and can become a specialist in his disease. It would be beyond the scope of this book to describe such details which are explained in books dealing specifically with this disease. In this chapter we shall relate only the criteria recommended by the Epidemiologic Society of Vienna in 1971 to evaluate blood sugar levels. The following table shows fasting levels as well as after meal glucose levels (determination of blood sugar is presented in mg%.)

| | | After Meal | |
	Fasting	One-Hour	Two-Hours
Normal	Under 100	under 160	under 120
Borderline	100-130	160-220	120-150
Pathological	above 130	above 220	above 150

Risk Factor: Elevated Uric Acid in the Blood (Hyperuricemia)

Dangers of gout

It has not been clearly determined whether this risk factor per se plays a significant role in coronary heart disease. However, this risk factor should be taken seriously since it is frequently found in association with other risk factors and, in addition, may lead to the development of other risk factors. The danger of hyperuricemia is demonstrated by the fact that coronary disease is three times as frequent in hypertensive patients with high uric acid levels as in hypertensives without hyperuricemia. The screening for elevated uric acid levels and gout should therefore be an integral part not only of high blood pressure treatment but also of every diagnostic work-up.

The upper normal limit for uric acid levels in the blood is 6mg%. It is advisable to bring patients with hyperuricemia exceeding 11mg% under treatment.

Risk Factor: Overweight

It is surprising that extensive surveys by epidemiologists have proven that overweight per se (without the interaction of the other risk factors hypercholesterolemia, hypertension, diabetes, gout, smoking) is not a risk factor for heart attacks. (However, overweight is a significant risk factor for angina pectoris because the frequency of angina pectoris is five times higher among obese patients than among persons with ideal weight.)

It is important to realize, however, that 85% of diabetics, 80% of persons with abnormal fat metabolism, 70% of patients with gout, and 60% of persons with high blood pressure are overweight. Thus weight loss is of utmost importance when related to these abnormal conditions.

Risk Factor: High Blood Pressure (Hypertension)

Although patients with hypertension do not experience discomfort in the early stages of the disease, one out of three patients dies as a result of it. It is indeed frightening for the cardiologist concerned with prevention to observe the grave consequence of a disease which is relatively easy to treat when diagnosed in the early stage. Statistics demonstrate that in the United States 15% of the adult population suffers from hypertension. Although, because of extensive media campaigns, many are now aware of their condition, far too few get proper treatment. As in all chronic diseases, the success of treatment depends to a large degree on the cooperation of the patient.

It is known that too few patients with hypertension take the prescribed medication regularly. Frequently drugs are taken so long as the symptoms of stroke and heart attack such as kidney or congestive heart failure persist. In such a case, however, it is often too late for effective treatment. But why are the statistics on *Hypertension—the silent threat* hypertension so discouraging? These statistics are the end-result of the fact that high blood pressure causes no complaints in the early stages and is therefore often neglected in contrast to low blood pressure which may show symptoms but is not fatal.

How can high blood pressure and its consequences be prevented? Everyone over 20 years of age should have his blood pressure checked annually. For adults the upper limit of normal blood pressure is 140/90 mm Hg. Unfortunately, cardiologists observe all too often that a patient with high blood pressure does not take his disease very seriously. We have therefore discussed hypertension extensively in this chapter. Since high blood pressure does not cause symptoms, the patient often takes the prescribed drugs only until the side effects such as fatigue and dizziness appear, although these result only because the blood pressure is lowered. These side effects would disappear within a short time period, but are regarded by the patient as poisonous. However, the side effects are not toxic, but instead are caused by the lowering of high blood pressure when the patient becomes temporarily hypotensive and experiences the complaints typical for a person with low blood pressure levels.

In view of the high incidence of hypertension and the underestimation of its consequences, we would like to ask you to consider whether one of your relatives or friends has high blood pressure. If at all possible try to urge a visit to a physician in order to discuss the problems of hypertension. You could possibly save a friend or relative from the long-term effects described.

Women who take the contraceptive pill are especially at high risk. For this reason the blood pressure of women who wish to take the pill is checked by the gynecologist.

Risk Factor: Cigarette Smoking

As early as 1965 the World Health Organization (WHO) stated explicitly what other epidemiological studies have proven so conclusively that no further studies are necessary: cigarette smoking is a major risk factor for coronary disease increasing in importance the younger the patient. The frequency of coronary disease is three times higher among cigarette smokers than it is among non- or ex-smokers, or non-inhaling pipe and cigar smokers. It is encouraging to note that cigarette smokers lower their risk of a heart attack within a few months after they quit smoking. Within a few years after they stop smoking, the risk of a heart attack is the same among ex-smokers and non-smokers. Dr. Nussel of the WHO study in Heidelberg discovered that the average age for the first heart attack is 63 for non-smokers, but 53 among smokers. According to the preliminary results of the Hohenrieder Myocardial Infarction Study, continued smoking is the most important risk factor for re-infarction and sudden death following a heart attack. Our youngest patient was only 17 years old and had smoked 3 packs a day.

Risk Factor: Lack of Exercise

Exercise as Prevention

The fact that physical inactivity still has not been proven conclusively to be a risk factor for coronary disease is probably due to the methodological problems involved in research, because it is difficult to define the extent of the need of exercise in each individual case. Occupations which involve sitting and passive leisure-time activities (such as sitting in front of the television or in bars) characterize a life-style in which the lack of exercise is clearly evident. There is, however, sufficient data available to indicate clearly that persons active in sports have a lower incidence of coronary disease and heart attacks. These data also demonstrate that persons active in sports are less prone to develop fatal complications in the first 48 hours following a heart attack.

Risk Factor: Hereditary Factors

Susceptibility to disease

It is very likely that hereditary factors play an important role in arteriosclerosis, hypertension, abnormal fat levels in the blood as well as in diabetes. However, it is difficult to establish in each individual case whether the major role is played by genuine genetic factors or so-called pseudo-genetic factors, such as poor living habits (for example, nutrition) from early childhood. There is no reason for resignation even in a family in which many risk factors are evident. Nevertheless, it is worthwhile to take great care in determining and treating all risk factors which are the result of a poor life-style, foremost among them smoking.

Risk Factor: Inflammations and Infections

It has yet to be proven that chronic inflammations are part of the risk factor profile, although certain studies show this result. Our youngest coronary infarction patient was an apprentice 17 years of age who not only smoked 3 packs a day, but also suffered from a urinary tract infection. This infection may have been an additional risk factor, because the heart attack occurred during the acute stage of his pyelitis. Similarly a patient with tonsillitis who mistreated his infection with sauna and running at the beach suffered a heart attack during the acute stage of his tonsillitis. Because of the possible role infection plays in heart attacks, we think that chronic inflammations (such as dental abscess, chronic tonsillitis, sinusitis, and gall bladder and kidney infections) should be treated immediately and vigorously.

Infections as a possible factor

Risk Factor: Contraceptive Pills

If a woman is not affected by any of the above mentioned risk factors it is very unlikely that the contraceptive pill per se will cause coronary heart disease or a heart attack. However, she does risk a heart attack if other risk factors are present and she takes the pill for several years. For this reason women consulting a gynecologist about the pill are checked for the presence of other risk factors such as hypertension, elevated cholesterol and triglyceride levels, as well as for smoking, overweight, and a positive family history. The combination of the pill with cigarette smoking is especially dangerous.

Risk Factor: Psycho-Social Stress and Risk Personality

Who is susceptible to stress?

When heart attack patients are asked what they believe caused their disease and this dramatic change in their life, half of the patients quickly respond. "Stress!" Is this reply a convenient excuse, a fashionable fatalistic attitude to avoid responsibility for one's life-style, or is stress a problem which we as physicians do not recognize as we should? Since these questions raise great doubt, we shall discuss this disputed problem in detail.

27

A person risks an early heart attack if his personality pattern belongs to Type A and is characterized in the following way: he cannot live without a clock, speaks in a hasty and abrupt manner, is unable to listen, constantly interrupts others, insists on doing several things simultaneously, focuses conversation on himself, constantly attempts to outdo others, cannot enjoy anything without a guilty conscience, clenches his fists, and skims over these lines with great impatience.

This description is quoted from the jacket of a Rowohlt book: *Type A and Type B* written by Doctors Meyer-Friedman and R.H. Rosenman (American edition: *Type A Behaviour and Your Heart,* Knopf, 1974). These two American physicians studied the behavior pattern of healthy individuals over several long term periods and subsequently differentiated two main types of behavior. They then compared the incidence of heart attack in the two groups, calling the description quoted above 'Type A' and the opposite of this personality pattern 'Type B'. After only a three year observation period, they discovered that the incidence of myocardial infarction was 2.2 times higher among individuals of Type A than among Type B. It must be added, however, that the findings of Meyer-Friedman and Rosenman are questioned in medical circles. Our opinion may be summarized with the following statement: although simplified, a coronary prone pattern (type A) behavior exists to some degree.

Primary risk factors

Many observers and epidemiologists express the opinion that the primary risk factors such as hypertension, abnormal fat metabolism, and smoking, have a common denominator in secondary risk factors. Thus there is in the view of some psychologists, sociologists, and animal experimentors a certain smoker's personality and a certain hypertensive life-style which leads to an increased activity of the sympathetic nervous system and thus to hypertension. In other words, the secondary risk factor is "stress." But what exactly do we mean by this?

Healthy stress and distress

Dr. H. Selye first defined stress as the reaction of an organism to external influences which provoke it to either fight or flight. Selye differentiates the life-preserving reaction as healthy stress (for example the immediate fight or flight reaction of a cat when it is provoked) from what he calls *distress* resulting from the impossibility of either fight or flight (as in the case of an imprisoned cat or man). However, this differentiation is not always valid in everyday situations. We therefore propose to make stress a more useful term by redefining it as over-exertion.

Almost half of our patients believed that stress in their occupation or personal life caused the heart attack. The patient apparently refers to over-exertion in his way of life which may have lasted for a long period of time and which resulted in disease when he was unable to resolve the problems. Scientists, in particular those involved in behavior modification and zoology, refer to this way of life as overloaded "role situations," which result for example when the normal social structure is altered. Dr. Lennart Levy in Stockholm has defined the following common stressors or psycho-social factors in over-exertion:

Psycho-social stressors

1) *Poor adjustment of people to their environment,* for example, discrepancies in occupation and personal life, between ability and capability, needs and possibilities, or expectations and reality.

2) *Over-exertion resulting from conflicting roles,* for example, in being both career-oriented and a family person.

3) *Problems due to the lack of life-fulfillment* which could sometimes be avoided, but cause crises, often in middle age, when we suddenly question the purpose of our existence.

4) *Frequent role changes,* for example, in occupation and place of living. This factor has been studied extensively and it has been shown that persons with greater mobility than others are more prone to heart attacks, although it has been questioned as a real contributing factor.

5) *Changes in social norms, institutions and roles* can be expressed in a more common manner as transformations of our values and attitudes in religion, marriage, partnership, authority and emancipation.

This list comprises the factors with which research is concerned, although it must be emphasized that the hypotheses mentioned are disputed by many physicians. It is also hoped that this discussion will enable the reader to evaluate his personal stress situation. Do you consider yourself as belonging to Type A described by Friedman and Rosenman? Are you excessively ambitious? Or can you identify with the following patient? A fifty year old owner of a small tool-making plant (25 employees) has been engaged in competitive sports since his youth, living in accordance with the point system established by the American sports physiologist, Dr.

Example of achievement stress

29

Cooper. He runs 12½ miles even on Christmas day and during his convalescence from a heart attack he measures the distance of one mile in order to run this exact distance back and forth at eight minutes per mile. Such exact measurements of time and distance are typical for this kind of person. But why does someone so active in sports sustain a heart attack? The probable answer is that he is excessively ambitious in both sports and his occupation. Nevertheless the fact that he was so active in sports prevented him form a more serious heart attack involving complications. It was only in the course of his convalescence that he realized he was 'programmed wrong' and should not be so extremely serious in all aspects of his life. Since the general interest in all aspects of psycho-social stress is wide-spread, we have described it in detail. An examination of personal stress and risk factors is helpful to each of us.

It follows from the discussion of the risk factors for coronary heart disease which have been established by new studies of epidemiologists, that metabolic as well as environmental factors must be detected and treated in an early stage. Furthermore, it is *A risk factor* clear that in the majority of cases no single risk factor, but instead *per se is rare* the interplay of various risk factors, causes the heart attack. Therefore all risk factors must be treated simultaneously in a comprehensive manner. Dr. Jahnecke, an experienced specialist of hypertension, draws the following analogy to emphasize the necessity of comprehensive treatment:

The elimination of one particular risk factor such as hypertension without concern for other risk factors is of little use. Similarly there is no sense in equipping a car with the newest safety belts but then speeding down the highway at night without lights, with worn-out tires and defective brakes.

What Are Your Personal Risk Factors?

By now it should be possible for you to apply the general information of this chapter in order to evaluate your personal risk profile by responding to the following questions:

1. Are your blood fat levels abnormal? More specifically, how

high is your cholesterol level? How high is your triglyceride level? Is your uric acid level elevated? When were these laboratory tests last done?

2. Are you overweight? What should your normal or ideal weight be (See chart, p.95)?
3. Do you have diabetes?
4. Is your blood pressure normal or elevated? When was it last checked?
5. Are you a cigarette smoker? How many cigarettes do you smoke per day? How long have you been smoking?
6. Do you exercise regularly? Would you describe your life-style as sports-oriented or not? For how many hours per week are you active in sports (for example, hiking, swimming, bicycle riding)? Less than two hours weekly?
7. Are you aware of any close relative (sisters and brothers, parents, grandparents) who sustained heart attacks, or have hypertension, diabetes, or abnormal fat levels (hypercholesterolemia)?
8. Do you suffer from any chronic infections? For example, sinusitis, chronic bronchitis, gall bladder or kidney infections (pyelitis)?
9. Do you think that you are under extreme psychological stress? Are you the extremely ambitious Type A personality described by Friedman and Rosenman?

The risk factors listed in these nine questions are by no means equally important or dangerous. For this reason we suggest that you do not evaluate your personal risk profile according to some kind of point system. Instead we believe that only a physician, familiar with your case history, is competent to explain the significance of various risk factors for you. Besides, only the risk factors mentioned in the first five questions are generally accepted, while questions six through nine are still in debate. The patient should be made aware of the controversial nature of some risk factors. We nevertheless emphasize that it may be of critical importance in certain cases to recognize and eliminate potentially harmful life-styles and habits whenever possible.

Can Heart Attacks and Re-Infarctions Be Prevented?

This question is crucial for the cardiologist, who must quote and rely on specialists, for example in life-table analysis. The head of the renowned Framingham Study, Dr. Kannel, replies to the question in this way: "We must advance to the point where we consider every heart attack to be a failure of preventive medicine." While this statement may be regarded as a mere dream for the future, it also provokes us to improve our preventive methods. Such questions are often raised at our congresses and force us to think about our responsibility to the patients. But often, Dr. Kannel's observation is misinterpreted as signifying that each and every heart attack could have been prevented. There are, of course, limits on the physician's influence: not only the personality of individual patients is to be considered, but even more importantly, their potential for changing their life-style. That is why our colleagues and the public often react with apathy.

Our experience in observing the process of coronary disease in thousands of patients over the years permits us to formulate the following answer to the lead question. Elimination or control of each of the previously discussed risk factors lowers the probability of a heart attack or its recurrence. Since modification of the life-style is almost always required, the saying that "man does not die as a result of his disease, but of his character," is true in many cases. A skeptical reader may suspect that the authors are embellishing the truth or are overly optimistic. Such a person has probably developed an attitude of resignation because of reading some statistics according to which the normal life-expectancy after a heart attack is limited to five years. But this particular statistic resembles the claim that a "normal" life-expectancy is seventy years of age (which is calculated by including infant morality and by placing greater emphasis on suicides and accidents of young persons, than on persons of one hundred years of age). Statistical interpretation must be weighed very carefully in the individual case.

The incidence of heart attacks or sudden death is higher in patients who have already sustained a myocardial infarction than in the general population. Dr. Ernest Wynder of the American Health Foundation once made a very appropriate statement: "We hope to die *young,* but as *late* as possible." Even a patient who suffers from coronary disease or has already sustained a heart attack can live a normal life both in terms of quality and normal life expectancy.

A colleague and friend of ours who is still active in sports had a heart attack when he was fifty-two years old. Despite this heart attack and subsequent irregular heart rhythm (atrial fibrillation) we found it difficult to follow him on a skiing tour high in the Alps when he was seventy-two years of age.

3. Cardio-Vascular Diagnostic Workshop

What Complaints and Symptoms May Indicate

"Everyone can take care of his own car. All that is needed is some interest in caring for it, as well as buying the necessary Volkswagen tools and carefully following our directions. Special maintenance, however, involves more than such care because it requires technical skills, workshop equipment and specific tools."

This text comes from a Volkswagen manual which is similar to the operating instructions of other cars. Careful reading reveals that a new car owner should have the routine maintenance done every ten thousand miles or at least once a year, and should not forget the lubrication and general maintenance required when car trouble develops.

Operating manual for your heart

Our book may be regarded as an "operating manual" for your heart, for what is good for your car should certainly be right for your heart. You should be reminded of having your cardio-vascular system checked, especially if you are middle-aged or when you develop certain symptoms and if you learn of a heart attack in your family.

What kind of tests should you anticipate when you visit your physician? Which kind of additional examinations are valuable? What is the potential outcome and prognosis of such examinations?

Three situations are possible:
• You have no complaints but would like to know whether you are as healthy as you feel.
• You do have complaints and would like to know whether you

suffer from ischemic heart disease. You would like to be informed on how such symptoms develop, what they signify and how they can be prevented.

● You have already sustained a heart attack and hope to prevent re-infarction.

If you have no complaints, you should continue your reading on page 41 where the actual physical examination is discussed.

Types and causes of symptoms

If, however, you still have complaints persisting since your first heart attack, then you are probably interested in finding out whether these symptoms originate in the heart or in another organ.

In any case, it is of utmost importance to you and your physician to find out the exact nature and causes of your symptoms. In 90% of the cases it is possible to determine the nature and cause of the symptom by questioning the patient. If you are interested in these questions, try to define and list your symptoms in the manner a physician would. The list on page 36 may serve as a guide.

This short questionnaire cannot, of course, replace the careful family and personal history established by a physician, but it can indicate the trend of your complaints if you respond consistently to either the questions on the right or on the left of the questionnaire. For example, if you responded to four or five questions on the left-hand side in the affirmative, then you must assume that your complaints are symptoms of a true angina pectoris and are warning signs of an imbalance between oxygen supply and demand of the heart muscle.

angina pectoris

As early as 1768, William Heberden, a famous English physician, described the symptoms in a manner which is still applicable today. "It is a pain which develops primarily after climbing stairs or eating, which can cause feelings of foreboding doom or even death and which ceases when standing still. The pain occurs when driving, riding a horse, swallowing, coughing, or during bowel movement, excitement, lying on the side and even while sleeping. The pain is localized under the breast bone, often more to the left than to the right, and can radiate to the arms and hands. It is not related to shortness of breath and usually affects only men . . . the chest-tightness caused by the pain may be referred to as 'angina pectoris' (chest-tightness)."

If you suspect that you are suffering from angina pectoris, you should consult your physician immediately, because your

35

List of Complaints
Self Testing for Patients

1. *Can you describe the nature of your complaints?*

Do you feel tightness, pressure, or heaviness but not a real pain and rarely combined with a feeling of fear?

Do you feel a stabbing or cutting pain or strong palpitations? Do you then experience difficulty with breathing?

2. *Can you describe the location of your pain?*

Do you feel tightness or pressure behind the breast bone, radiating to the throat, teeth, stomach, between the shoulder blades, in one or both arms?

Do you feel the stabbing or cutting pain directly in the heart region so that you can point to it with your finger? Is the skin directly over the heart sensitive to pressure?

3. *Which situations trigger your symptoms?*

Quick physical activities such as walking or climbing stairs? Especially on a cold morning? After heavy meals?

Changing weather conditions? Emotional stress and excitement? Certain movements?

4. *Can you describe the length or duration of your symptons?*

Do tightness and pressure last a few minutes?

Do your complaints last for a few seconds? Or are they of longer duration?

5. *How can you influence your complaints?*

By immediately stopping all activity and resting?

By moving around a little and perhaps getting a breath of fresh air?

complaints are probably caused by a narrowing of the coronary vessels. This narrowing of the blood vessels—actually arteriosclerosis of the coronary vessels—can lead to shortage of blood and oxygen supply. Thus, the demand of oxygen in the heart during physical exercise, under time-pressure or after a heavy meal, cannot be met.

This description holds true for all patients who have sustained a heart attack and experience further symptoms. (A few people with a problem involving the valves of the heart may have chest pain with normal coronary arteries. They are in no danger of heart attack and they require a different type of treatment.)

Suspected diagnosis: "dyscardia"

If, however, you responded in the affirmative to most of the questions on the right-hand side of the questionnaire, then the probable diagnosis is "dyscardia". This term refers to pain in the left chest which is differentiated from true angina pain in location, duration, precipitation and possible alleviation. "Dyscardia" is caused neither by narrowing of coronary vessels, nor by an insufficient oxygen supply to the myocardium.

The spinal column can cause heart complaints

Experience has shown that such chest pains occur not only as a result of impaired circulation, but also in arthritic changes in the vertebrae of the neck or chest or even in the muscles of the chest wall and in the ribs where they join the breast bone. These complaints are also common in vertebral column complications causing pain in the arms, neck and shoulder. Usually the symptoms in the left chest cease when the complications involving the vertebral column have disappeared. Using X-rays the physician often detects changes in the spinal cord (degenerative changes) possibly combined with muscle cramps or functional difficulties. The patients are commonly under forty and those with "dyscardia" are mostly women, while those suffering from angina are predominately men.

If the spinal column is the cause of the symptoms, the complaints usually occur when the head is held in a certain position, for example, when sleeping with a poor posture. The complaints disappear when the position is altered, after loosening up exercises, or gymnastics. These pseudo-heart symptoms must be treated in the same manner in which all complications originating in the vertebral column are treated, through prevention of great strain (long hours of uninterrupted typing, driving, or sewing), with relaxing exercises (morning gymnastics, walking or sports) and something which is typically taught in European spas,

37

climate-therapy (alternating hot and cold showers, sauna, etc.). This program may be supplemented by massages of the connective tissues, use of heat, chiropractic measures and electrotherapy.

It is possible to differentiate radiating pain which is a result of vertebral complications from that resulting from angina pectoris. Complications involving the vertebral column cause pain which typically radiates into the outer side of the arms and which occurs in certain positions, while true heart pain radiates into the inner sides of the arms and increases in intensity with exertion. Pain resulting from vertebral column complications is often felt in the right thumb, while heart pain radiates to the left small and ring fingers. Moreover, complications involving the vertebral column can be distinguished from those involving the heart by the use of medication. Ask your physician for a nitroglycerin capsule and bite the capsule to release its fluid the next time you feel the heart pain. If the capsule does not alleviate your pain then you are probably suffering from "dyscardia".

Testing with a nitro capsule

"Heart" pains may originate not only in the vertebral column, but may also be caused by "nerves" or emotional stress. This type of pain is more frequent among young people, usually under the age of forty, than among older persons, and is also found more among women than men. Intense chest pain may be experienced, although no disease is detectable in the coronary vessels. In such a case, there is nothing wrong with the patient's heart. These complaints are sometimes referred to as "heart neurosis" when diagnostic procedures give no evidence of actual disease.

Heart complaints and nerves

Of the patients suffering from heart trouble, 30% to 40% have a non-organic, so-called nervous dysfunction of the cardio-vascular system which appears to be a problem in the heart. Careful examinations of the duration and causes of the complaints can help in differential diagnosis according to the situation which triggered the chest pain:

● Confrontation with an accident, illness or death which involves heart problems on the part of others.
● Disturbing warning signs.
● Emotional conflicts.

Since the physical symptoms do not always appear directly after the emotional event, the patient usually does not associate his physical with his emotional complaints. It is now known that pseudo-cardiac disorders are usually caused by the trauma of separation. Dr. W. Brautigam explains: "If we examine the

38

situation of the patient at the onset of his disease, we find that nearly all are characterized by a conflict of separation. The majority of patients were involved in an internal or external conflict with a mother figure at that time." Dr. H. E. Richter confirms " . . . that the onset of the disease coincides with a threat to a protective and dependent relationship the patient had cultivated. The 'heart neurosis' manifests itself at a time when either the patient or the other person involved in the relationship withdraws or threatens the relationship. . . . The actual dilemma for the patient is that he unconsciously revolts against his dependence on the relationship but fears destruction without it. The patient who often becomes sick when he feels he could become more independent is actually already more independent. It is as if he were being punished for seeking or attaining independence from a person to whom he had been closely tied. This punishment makes the patient even more helpless and impotent." Richter describes very typical examples of such a situation: A thirteen year old boy has a very domineering and overly protective mother. He experiences his first attack when he joins a friend on a bicycle tour from which his mother had tried to discourage him. At twenty-four years of age he experiences a further series of dyscardic attacks when the occasion of an examination allows him to leave his home.

A few typical examples

A twenty year old nurse visits her parents over Christmas. The visit culminates in a misunderstanding which is not resolved. After her departure she waits in vain for letters from her mother who had always corresponded regularly. As a result she develops dyscardic symptoms.

A thirty year old married patient is unfaithful. Although he feels very close to his wife, whom he regards as a kind of mother figure, he is strongly attracted to another woman. He also develops dyscardic symptoms.

In the event that you did not determine any risk factors in your case and responded positively to the questions on the right hand side of the questionnaire at the beginning of this chapter, answer the questions which concern the symptoms of dyscardia (see box, page 40).

It is possible that you have dyscardia if you answered more than half of the questions with "often" and, in addition, frequently feel fatigued, experience shortness of breath, feel trembling, faintness or weakness in your legs and arms, have insomnia and

Conflicts caused by separation

39

Accompanying symptoms	often	rarely	never
Are you depressed?	☐	☐	☐
Are you anxious without cause or reason?	☐	☐	☐
Do you have a tendency to overprotect yourself both emotionally and physically?	☐	☐	☐
Are you restless?	☐	☐	☐
Do you often experience palpitations?	☐	☐	☐
Do you fear that you suffer from coronary disease?	☐	☐	☐
Are you afraid of heart attack?	☐	☐	☐

experience abdominal and intestinal discomfort. We have described dyscardic symptoms in detail since thay may also appear after an actual heart attack. Not all complaints experienced after a heart attack can be attributed to attacks of angina pectoris and it is even possible to suffer from anginal pain and "dyscardia" simultaneously. These symptoms often persist stubbornly and torment the patient without involving actual changes in blood vessel walls. During the treatment which should proceed with patience, the emotional state must be determined. Patients suffering from both angina and "dyscardia" should be treated with graded exercise (see pages 108-110) and possibly hydrotherapy as well as with an appropriate diet. The two types of patients should be distinguished only in drug therapy, although beta blockers (see page 89) are helpful in treating both angina and "dyscardia".

Discussing the findings with your doctor

After the physician determines your symptoms by questioning you carefully, he will try to establish your risk profile as you did yourself in the section entitled "Your Personal Risk Factors". He will ask about your smoking and eating habits, your work, possible stress situations in your profession and family, and also about how you relax.

Establishing the medical history

Questions about sports, hobbies and your spare-time activities form an integral part of the case-history. Hereditary factors must also be determined as part of the personal history. Typical questions include the age at death of your parents and the incidence of heart attack, stroke, hypertension, diabetes, gout and abnormal fat levels in the blood among close relatives. Is your family overweight, or normal weight, or thin?

Computerized
questionnaires

Do not be surprised if you must answer these questions on a lengthy and possibly computerized form. Your physician uses these carefully developed forms not only to save time but also to attain a higher degree of diagnostic accuracy. This way the physician is able to make a preliminary diagnosis which he will substantiate in the course of his conversation with you.

The Physical Examination

The physician examines your heart by determining the rhythm and frequency of the heart rate. A normal pulse lies between 60 and 100 heart beats per minute. An irregular heart rate is called "arrhythmia" and extra heart beats are "extra-systolic". Moreover, he checks the opening and closing functions of the heart valves with the stethoscope because the valves may have been damaged by scars (valve defects). Valve defects caused by scars can be detected by the abnormal sounds they make. However, it is impossible to detect sure signs of coronary sclerosis, impaired circulation to the heart muscle, or a previous heart attack by using a stethoscope. For this reason EKG's must be taken.

The next step in the physical examination is to listen to the lungs because the heart may be strained (decompensated) as in congestive heart failure and as a result of chronic bronchitis from cigarette smoking (with pulmonary emphysema caused by a loss of elasticity of the small air sacs—alveoli which are located at the end of the air tubes).

Determining
arterial
changes

The general state of the cardio-vascular system may indicate the condition of your heart. Arteriosclerotic changes in the arteries of the body, for example, of the feet and ankles, may be determined by taking the pulse which, in the case of arteriosclerosis is very weak or absent. Listening to the abdominal aorta may reveal loud bruits, indicating atherosclerotic changes and severe thinning of the aortic walls, a so-called aneurysm.

The blood pressure reading is of particular importance (see page 24 under Risk Factors). Moreover the correct relationship between

41

height and weight is determined for the individual case (see page 94). At the same time a blood sample is taken in order to obtain the cholesterol, triglyceride, blood sugar and uric acid levels (see pages 20-23).

EKG at Rest and Work (Bicycle Ergometry)

What kind of information does a physician receive from an EKG, and how is an EKG made? The EKG is a routine procedure which is frequently used, the results of which can be partially evaluated by a computer, but are often overestimated. Sometimes patients fear the EKG because they are under the false impression that electrical currents are sent through their bodies. What really happens?

How is an EKG made?

Each heart beat produces a very weak electrical current of .001 volts. Highly sensitive instruments can measure these currents in the arms, legs, and chest by amplifying the signals and then measuring them. It is even possible to make EKG's without using any wires connecting to the patient.

Abnormal waves often indicate impaired circulation of the heart muscle resulting from, for example, coronary arteriosclerosis or a heart attack. It is also feasible to detect an abnormal rhythm. Unfortunately, it is not possible to state with absolute certainty from a normal EKG that a heart is healthy. In fifty percent of coronary patients, the EKG at rest does not show significant abnormality!

EKG at rest is not sufficient

For this reason, the physician will also order an exercise EKG if he suspects coronary heart disease. This EKG is made while the patient walks on a treadmill or sits pushing the peddles of an exercise bicycle. Depending upon the peddle resistance, the patient can achieve twenty-five, fifty, seventy-five or a hundred watts of work energy. At the same time the pulse rate and blood pressure are monitored. Following the procedure of exercise, the recuperation capacity is evaluated as the body returns to the resting state. The EKG may also be observed by a wireless (telemetric) EKG during an exercise therapy session as in the course of rehabilitation from a heart attack. Recently an EKG has

Treadmill EKG

been developed in the form of a small box which the patient carries for a twenty-four hour period. In this manner, abnormal and possibly dangerous aberrations of the heart rhythm can be detected if it is suspected that a certain daily activity causes problems for the patient.

Bicycle ergometry or treadmill EKG's can be very useful. Impaired circulation of the myocardium, the effect of medication, as well as abnormal rhythm not discoverable by a resting EKG can thus be detected and treated in an early stage. Moreover, bicycle ergometry can be used for training in the rehabilitation after a heart attack.

Fluoroscopy and X-Rays

Information about the heart and lungs

Information concerning the heart and lungs can be gained from fluoroscopy and chest X-rays. The size and form of the heart (ventricles, aorta and auricles) are of particular interest, because enlarged auricles and ventricles indicate an overburdened and congested, decompensated heart muscle. It is not difficult to detect calcification of the valves, heart sac (pericardium), and aorta, or fluid in the lungs, both of which indicate that the heart is weakened. The success of the therapy may be measured by comparing these films to later X-rays. A patient who looks at a chest X-ray for the first time can easily recognize the vertebral column and ribs, but is likely to be disappointed when he tries to identify the heart, because it does not resemble the idealized form found in love letters. The heart as seen on an X-ray is simply a dense white shadow or sac without definite contours.

Special Examinations

Coronary angiography

Dr. Werner Forssmann made it possible to gain more information from X-rays of the heart when he developed a method of inserting a thin catheter into the vein of the arm and pushing it toward the heart. He experimented on himself in 1929 and received the Nobel Prize in 1946 for this method. It is feasible to observe more details

*The heart
seen on a
special film*

in the X-ray films made by this method because a contrast fluid can be injected through the catheter and into the coronary vessels of the heart (a process called coronary angiography). Thus, coronary artery blockages could be identified and it could be determined how well the blood flows through the coronaries. Great advances have been made since 1970 in developing so-called invasive diagnosis, especially in coronary angiography, to evaluate the function of the heart muscle and the coronary arteries. It is now regarded as merely a routine procedure, which has passed successfully through the experimental stage and is used in most large hospitals.

Coronary angiography is used more frequently as, for example, to determine whether surgery is required in the case of a patient who experiences intense pain caused by angina pectoris which cannot be alleviated through medication. In such cases it is often possible to relieve the chest pain by performing a by-pass operation (see page 73).

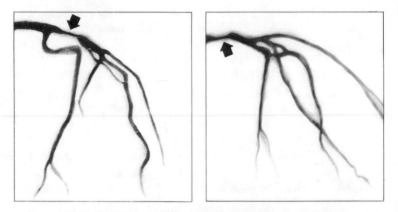

These drawings show how coronary vessels filled with contrast medium appear on an X-ray. The arrows point to vessel changes. (The drawings are based on X-rays.)

*Small risk
and great
benefit*

But is a coronary angiography not harmful to a patient with a damaged heart? Of course, such invasive diagnostic procedures can cause undesirable side effects but usually only one out of two thousand patients develops such complications in cardiology departments with experienced personnel. Since it is virtually impossible to obtain the vital information on the condition of the

44

coronary vessels by any other means (an EKG yields only indirect information), we must rely upon angiography even though it involves relatively small risks.

If you are a patient before or after a heart attack you will probably respond with mixed feelings to the news that this procedure needs to be carried out. The thought of coronary angiography will probably make you uneasy or perhaps afraid, feelings which are to be expected. But what is involved in this procedure? What will you actually feel? In our experience, a conversation with someone who has already undergone angiography is much more valuable than any written explanatory statement by a physician. Do you know such a patient personally? If not, you could ask your physician to acquaint you with someone who has experienced a coronary angiography. If you are uneasy or afraid, you can also request special medication to ease discomfort.

Talk with
other patients

The procedure is as follows. The point at which the catheter will be inserted is either in the main artery on the inside of the thigh or the artery inside the elbow. This point of entry is usually anesthetized, and if the injection into the large vessel causes discomfort, you can request another local anesthetic, as you would ask a dentist during tooth work. A special catheter is inserted via the artery into the aorta and to the heart. An X-ray contrast medium is then injected through the catheter into the right and left coronary arteries. This part of the process is completely painless and the angiogram is recorded on film. The film will yield important information about the blood supply to the heart and the condition of the coronary vessels. Thereafter, more contrast fluid is injected into the ventricle (ventriculography) to determine the size and functioning of the heart and how well it contracts. Finally the catheter is removed and a compression bandage is placed over the point at which the catheter was introduced. The less bleeding occurs, the smaller will be a bruise mark in the thigh or arm, depending on the insertion location. After reading the films, three possible results may be discussed with the patient.

A painless
procedure

First Finding:
Operation not
necessary

1. It may be decided that an aorta-coronary by-pass operation (involving the aorta and coronary vessels) is unnecessary. In this case, you will certainly be relieved. This will be the case if the coronary arteries are completely free of blockages or if it is only a matter of the normal aging process. Or it may be that certain changes have taken place in the vessel walls but that they cause

45

the patient no discomfort, so an operation is unwarranted. As a matter of fact, half of the persons between ages fifty and sixty develop certain coronary atherosclerotic changes, but the narrowing of the vessels is not always sufficiently significant to require surgery.

Second Finding: Surgery recommended
2. The cardiologist recommends surgery, because coronary angiography has revealed a critical narrowing, for example, in the main trunk of the left coronary artery. It is the opinion of most surgeons that the survival rate of such patients with surgery is higher than that of those who do not receive an operation. In this case the patient must consider whether he should eliminate his risk by having the operation done, even if he does not experience great discomfort at that time. If, however, the patient does experience great chest pain from angina pectoris, then the cardiologist and cardiac surgeon may share the opinion that surgery will relieve the pain more quickly than would prologed drug therapy. The cardiologist will then explain to the patient whether a one, two or three vessel by-pass is indicated. The patient may have little choice but to accept the surgery, because if he delays too long, a second coronary angiography may become necessary (see page 73 for details of the by-pass operation).

Another type of surgery may be indicated after a heart attack. Ventriculography (which reveals the capacity of the heart to pump blood) may show a disrupted movement of the walls of the ventricles, usually caused by scar tissue from a previous heart attack. Some patients do not remember that they have sustained a heart attack, but the disrupted movement of the ventricular walls shows evidence of myocardial infarction.

In the scar area, an aneurysm or sac, formed by local softening and thinning of the arterial wall, may develop. This certainly interferes with the normal cardiac rhythm or may cause complications leading to heart failure and formation of blood clots. It is extremely rare that such an aneurysm will burst. If an aneurysm has developed, then a bulge in the vessel wall will be visible during ventriculography. In the contraction or systolic phase, the shadow of the injected contrasting material is greater in the area of the aneurysm, while this usually decreases in a healthy heart. In such cases, surgery is often recommended to remove the aneurysm (see page 75).

Third Finding: Surgery not recommended
3. The third possibility is that heart surgery at its present stage may be judged to be of no greater benefit than prolonged drug

treatment (page 86, "Long-Term Drug Therapy"). If the narrowing of the vessel wall is in the periphery of the myocardium, the vessels are too small for surgery. Very small, thin by-passes do not remain open for very long, so the operation would have no long-term success. However, it is very likely that such technical problems will be resolved in the near future.

It is known that by-pass operations can alleviate the chest pain resulting from angina, but researchers are not certain whether they increase the length of life. A patient who expects miraculous results from surgery in this age of technology, instead of making small preventive efforts, can often be disappointed. The patient

Overestimat-ing surgery

who tends to overrate surgery, underestimate non-surgical procedures, and who counts on the immediate success of surgery is equally dismayed. Although we can sympathize with such disappointment, we cannot share it, since there are many non-surgical procedures described in this book which can help resolve many problems. Even a successful by-pass operation is only a small part of a comprehensive plan for treatment. Although surgery enriches the possibilities for treatment of chronic heart disease, it is certainly not a universal remedy.

Swan Gans catheter
This diagnostic procedure involves no risk, little intervention and requires only devices which are available in an ordinary hospital. The examination may be repeated several times and yields important information, especially when combined with the previously described ergometry including the EKG.

How the procedure is done

The procedure consists of several steps. First, a thin two-way catheter within a special needle is inserted into a locally anesthetized arm vein. A tiny, thin expandable balloon is at the tip of the catheter. Once in the vein, the catheter flows with the blood stream into the right auricle, and through the right ventricle into the pulmonary artery. The patient cannot feel this movement during the procedure. The end of the catheter outside the arm is attached to a transducer. This tiny instrument changes the fluid pressure inside the right auricle, the ventricle and the pulmonary artery into an electrical impulse which is then recorded. An EKG is done simultaneously with the pressure measurements.

After measuring these values at rest, the patient takes the bicycle ergometer test. The EKG, heart rate, blood pressure and the fluid pressure of pulmonary circulation are measured and registered continuously.

When the findings of the usual examinations do not reveal any alterations, elevated pressure readings of pulmonary circulation can be the first signs of a heart attack. No other method is available to detect weakening in the pumping action of the heart in the early stages of heart disease. Moreover, it is possible to judge the effectiveness of medication and the way in which it affects the tolerance for physical exertion. After the examination, the catheter is removed and the point of injection is covered with a bandage, so the patient can return to his normal activities.

Heart scintiscan

This method is like the scintiscan of other organs, and is a relatively new and simple method of examination which yields a great deal of information. However, it is usually performed only in specialized medical centers.

A non-invasive procedure

This so-called "non-invasive" procedure does not cause any discomfort. The patient can feel only the injection of a small amount of radioactive tracer material into a vein of his arm. He is then placed under a highly sensitive instrument that detects the radioactivity and converts it into a film.

There are two basic methods for heart scintiscan. One method involves radioactive tracers which accumulate in healthy areas of the heart muscle with a sufficient blood supply, but not in the diseased areas with insufficient supply. The radioactive tracers do not accumulate in the diseased areas, because of insufficient blood supply. One such tracer is thallium which has biological features similar to potassium. The second method uses pyrophosphate which accumulates in the opposite manner in diseased tissue affected by heart attack, but not in the healthy "hot" areas.

Either way, the accumulation or lack of these materials can indicate on the film those areas in which the blood supply is insufficient and can reveal the actual size of a myocardial infarct.

The patient cannot feel the radiography as the plate registers the radioactive rays and converts them into a visible image. Thus the process may be repeated as many times as is necessary without causing the patient any discomfort. The method is time-consuming, however, because the patient must lie under the radiographic instrument during a second examination to determine the capacity of the heart to pump blood. In the treatment of coronary heart disease and myocardial infarction, the capacity of the heart to pump blood as well as its functioning and vigor are as important as the coronary circulation. The next step is to examine the ventricles, an examination which resembles the previous heart scintiscan. Radioactive albumin, which is injected before and after contraction, is detectable by radiographic instruments and converted into a radiographic image.

Ventricles are visualized

Since both scintiscans must be done from different angles of viewing, the procedure requires about one hour. The examination also requires that the patient fast prior to the procedure because digestive metabolism alters the biological distribution of thallium during scintiscan of the heart muscle. Since this procedure uses radioactive materials, the patient invariably raises questions about exposure, as he should. The radioactive exposure resulting from this procedure yields information about the heart that no other method can yield and the exposure is no greater than that of usual X-ray film processes. The scintiscan can be applied not only at rest, but also after physical activity, so that it is possible to determine the reaction of a damaged heart muscle to physical strain. It is also important to note that this examination can be performed on seriously ill patients following a recent heart attack. Another advantage is that the scintiscan allows determination of the location and size of a heart attack in the early stage; that is, when signs of the heart attack are not yet evident, in blood enzymes or in the EKG. A third advantage is that the examination can be repeated any time in order to carefully observe and monitor the course and progression of coronary heart disease.

Determining the location and size of the heart attack

Echo-cardiography

This modern diagnostic procedure which is also known as ultrasound cardiography is even more convenient for the patient than the previously described heart scintiscan. Ultrasound waves are sound waves which are too high in frequency to be detected by the human ear (limited to 20 kilohertz) and are used not only in technology and medicine, but also by bats. Bats are blind and orient themselves using ultrasound in their search for insects. In order to navigate, the bat emits ultrasound waves and then senses the echoes of these waves from objects which reflect them back to the bat.

Diagnosis through ultrasound waves

Ultrasound waves were first used in technology to locate submarines and schools of fish (echo sounder) or to detect small structural defects in materials.

One of the main reasons for using ultrasound in both technology and medicine is that these waves (unlike those which can be heard by the human ear) can be "bundled" easily. They are also governed by familiar optical laws of reflection and refraction. Moreover, ultrasound waves are reflected by very small objects and surfaces, since they have a relatively short wavelength.

In ultrasound cardiography (UCG) the sound waves are generated by a transducer which also receives the echoes of the waves. The high frequency sound waves are produced by a piezoelectric crystal to which a high-frequency alternating current is applied, causing the crystal to vibrate in rhythm with it. The patient does not feel the ultra-sound as it is directed toward the heart, reflected, and its echo returns to the piezoelecric crystal, which is mechanically distorted. The sound energy is converted into electric energy and the resulting electrical voltage may be represented visually on an oscilloscope. From this image, the

Drawing conclusions

technician can draw conclusions about the structure of the heart muscle, the atria ventricles, the pericardium and even the cardiac valves. This non-invasive technique for diagnosis can also be repeated at any time.

Thus the physician or heart specialist has a wide range of diagnostic tools at his disposal to examine heart disease in great detail.

Discussion of the Results of an Examination

Of what use is the best diagnosis if the patient:
- does not learn the results?
- does not understand the results?
- does not understand the necessary consequences?

Understanding the results of an examination

This aspect of the patient-physician relationship is one of great importance. It is, however, not different from other misunderstandings in human relationships. As physicians we often assume too hastily that our explanations have been understood. If the patient does not follow our advice, we react with disappointment, anger or resignation. From the physician's point of view, what can the patient do to improve this situation? First of all, you, the patient, must ask questions in order to understand the findings of the examination. It is likely that you must overcome various inhibitions such as fear of being obtrusive, of being turned away, or being told that the physician is too busy, or of appearing stupid if you cannot understand the explanation offered. Perhaps your physician is not fully aware of your interest in understanding your own disease. If this is the case, it may be possible for him to discuss the findings of the examination with you after his office hours. You would perhaps be well-advised to acquaint yourself with medical terminology and insights before your consultation by reading a book such as this one.

The following story may help you to overcome your fears and to ask additional questions when you do not understand the explanations. Several years ago, the author was walking with a patient who was also a tax consultant, and who had recently sustained a heart attack. For two hours the tax consultant patiently tried to explain to the doctor the nature of her tax return, while she listened attentively but was unable to understand the explanations. After a while the roles were reversed and the doctor tried to explain to the tax consultant what caused his heart attack, what it meant, and why he should undertake certain steps as a remedy. Both noticed after a while they had fallen silent and were walking next to each other perplexed. The tax consultant was the first to admit that he had not understood the detailed and interesting account his physician had presented. He felt the doctor had attempted to inform him of something very important, but it was impossible for him to understand the explanations since they were expressed in medical terminology. So they began again and each tried to explain to the other as a teacher would explain new material to a student with greater attention to the other's abilities and experiences. Thus the conversation came to a happy conclusion.

4. The Impending Heart Attack and the Acute Stage

The First Signs of a Heart Attack.

In obituaries of daily newspapers phrases such as the following are frequently found: "Suddenly while at work" or "In the midst of his creative period the fifty-two year old N. M. sustained a heart attack." But does this event occur unexpectedly, without any warning? "Did you not feel any pain prior to the heart attack?" the anxious relatives ask the patient in the intensive care unit. This question actually presupposes another one. Could the heart attack have been averted either by long-term prevention or immediate action prior to the attack, if certain symptoms had been taken more seriously?

Does a heart attack really come "out of the blue"? A study at the University Clinic in Heidelberg appears to corroborate this assumption, because of 913 coronary patients, 38% felt no symptoms four weeks prior to the heart attack. However, 30% of those who developed a heart attack, did notice certain warning signs.

Warnings which may indicate an impending heart attack include the following:

Signs of an impending heart attack

- Chest pain (debilitating pain in the left chest) which the patient has never felt before, and
- Changes in an already diagnosed angina pectoris. The pain becomes more frequent and intense, and of longer duration.

In this stage the physician must be consulted immediately and the patient must clearly describe the new chest pains or changes in the previously diagnosed disease. Only when the physician hears a detailed account, can he determine the danger of an impending heart attack and decide which steps should be taken to prevent it.

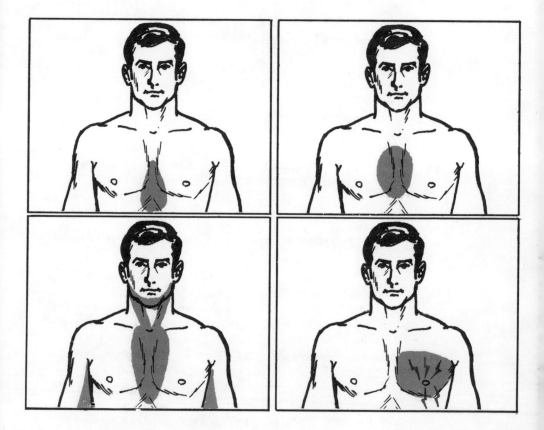

1. The normal position of the heart within the chest, behind the breast bone. **2.** Radius of the characteristic chest pain in patients suffering from angina pectoris, extending from behind the breast bone into the left and right chest. **3.** Different locations of warning signals for an impending myocardial infarct or the typical places where pain may occur in the initial phase of a heart attack. Usually the chest pain is limited to the heart behind the breast bone, radiating in the left arm. However it is entirely possible that also the right arm is involved or only the right arm may be involved. The pain is only rarely radiating into the neck and into the lower jaw. However, there have been patients who have gone to their dentists because of an intensive pain in the lower jaw where X-rays showed no abnormalities and only then the correct diagnosis was made by an electrocardiogram. **4.** A numb feeling in the left chest, sometimes mild stabbing pains usually in connection with emotional upheavals or excitement are not typical for heart attacks. The decision is usually made by the electrocardiogram. *(S. Heyden)*

He may decide to hospitalize the patient for rest, or to reduce risk factors and the danger of blood clotting or he may decide that an angiocardiogram is necessary.

Unfortunately, only a small number of those who notice the symptoms described previously, actually consult the physician before it is too late.

Is it possible to go directly to the hospital without first consulting the physician? Since this question is often posed in patient discussion groups, we shall answer it now in the affirmative: if a heart attack or re-infarction is suspected, the patient can enter the hospital directly and must be treated.

Go to a hospital immediately!

Symptoms of the Acute Stage

Symptoms of a heart attack

The major symptom of heart attack is severe and prolonged chest pain (angina pectoris). This agonizing feeling of pressure, chest tightness, and cutting pain may be new and alarming to the patient and may radiate into both arms, the abdomen, or the area between the shoulder blades. Other patients experience and describe a burning sensation behind the breast bone which extends to the neck or even the teeth of the lower jaw. Patients with chronic angina pectoris or who have sustained a heart attack previously are familiar with the pain which becomes increasingly intense and more prolonged prior to the actual heart attack.

The "silent" heart attack

Additional symptoms which accompany those previously mentioned are somewhat more difficult to describe, but are easily recognized. The patient's face is almost transfigured, is of pale or gray color, with an anxious expression; perspiration appears profusely and he is restless, short of breath, or breathes only superficially and avoids exerting himself. Other signs include vomiting, urgent need for bowel movement, fear of destruction, and mortal dread. "Silent" heart attacks with few or no symptoms are also possible, especially in older patients or those with diabetes. These "silent" heart attacks are often discovered merely by chance when the causes for severe shortness of breath and inability to exert oneself are closely examined.

Two heart attack patients tell their stories

The following two case histories related by the patients themselves are typical:

T.R., forty-eight years of age, a salesman, recalls: "I have

54

always been very healthy and have been able to work very hard. Once a year my wife would send me to the doctor because she thought I smoked too much. He always told me the same thing, that I should smoke less, although my EKG was normal. Since my blood pressure was a little too high, he once prescribed certain drugs, but they did not help. They made me tired, so I finally stopped taking them. On the day of the heart attack I was driving on the highway in the rain. Suddenly, I felt a pulling pain in my left arm and had a feeling of tightness in my chest, which I could not localize. I was covered with perspiration, had difficulty breathing, and became nauseous. Then I felt pain in my heart. Something was wrong with it, because I could sense extra beats and it seemed to be unsteady like a car engine that has problems with the ignition. I drove to a parking lot to breathe deeply and wait for this nonsense to stop. Nausea and a cramp in my esophagus made me think that I had an upset stomach or that I had been driving too long. Since I thought fresh air would make me feel better I did a few push-ups on the parking lot in the rain, but physical exertion made the pain worse. I do not remember how I managed to drive home. My wife was shocked. She must have realized that I was gravely ill because she drove me directly to the hospital without first calling the doctor. And now I am here having sustained an anterior wall infarction."

He should have known better

R. B., fifty-two years old, and a veterinarian, should have known better: "I had sustained a heart attack two years ago and had recovered quickly from it. I had no complaints whatsoever a year and a half later. But then I had attacks of angina pectoris again, at first only after heavy meals and when I had over-exerted myself. Right before the heart attack I no longer felt well, did not move very much, and regained the eighteen pounds I had lost. When I had these attacks with a feeling of pressure in my chest and the radiating pain between my shoulder blades and in my abdomen, I did not tell my wife because I did not want to worry her. I only told her when the attacks became more frequent, almost daily, before the heart attack and when my wife noticed that I needed more nitro capsules. But one night the nitro capsules did not alleviate the pain and I had terrible pains in my stomach, which made me think that I had a peptic ulcer. However, we did not call the doctor until the next afternoon. He knew immediately what was wrong and had me hospitalized. In the meantime I felt extremely weak and my pulse dropped to fifty beats per minute. The diagnosis was a posterior wall infarction."

Warning signs ignored

What conclusions can be drawn from these two case histories? In the case of a heart attack without pain prior to it, the heart attack can be predicted only by examining the different risk factors which exist simultaneously. In this case, both smoking and high blood pressure were present. If the patient does experience chest pain, then it is conceivable that the physician and the patient could cooperate in recognizing the danger and preventing the heart attack. However, the patient who is in danger of re-infarction often ignores warning symptoms because he refuses to believe that they are real. The veterinarian allowed fifteen hours to pass before he allowed his wife to call the doctor. During those fifteen hours outside the hospital, he was in constant danger to his life.

The Dangers of the First Hours

Statistical studies show that the most crucial phase from the onset of the symptoms to the contact with a physician lasts an average of three to seven hours. As a result of technical advances and progress in drug therapy, the mortality rate of acute heart attacks in the hospital has been reduced to one-half of the original rate in the last few years. However, a majority of patients with heart

Quick help is crucial

attacks die outside the hospital. Therefore, it would be best if the physician could reach the patient as soon as possible in the earliest phase of the acute heart attack. The patient should be brought to the hospital, preferably to the intensive care unit if it is at all possible to transport him. In the early phase of the heart attack, any number of serious complications can arise which require all the technical assistance and skilled personnel the clinic can muster. The family doctor simply cannot prevent and treat dangerously abnormal heart rhythm, shock, and cardiac insufficiency in the private home.

Critical period of decision-mak-ing

How can this critical period of decision-making between the first symptoms, the contact with the physician, and hospitalization be reduced? Presumably by means of education through mass media (or by reading this book) in order to make everyone aware of the symptoms of an impending heart attack. However, it has

56

happened that patients with symptoms of dyscardia (see page 37) are rushed to the hospital in ambulances for no good reason. But in such a case, it is necessary to determine the lesser of two evils. Is it not better to sound the alarm for ten different suspected cases of heart attack which are actually not serious, than to forego a life-saving chance one time when it is crucial?

What Can Relatives Do If a Heart Attack Is Suspected?

What should husbands or wives do if they realize that their spouse is threatened by a heart attack? Spouses of someone who is at risk repeatedly ask this question of their physician. They are motivated by the understandable fear that they may neglect to take a certain life-saving measure or that they may even do something wrong. That is why in our Hohenried Clinic and elsewhere, the Red Cross teaches courses in resuscitation so spouses of the heart attack patient may also participate. Even if the person cannot employ the techniques on a spouse, the techniques may be able to save the life of another person.

Tips for the spouse
We would now like to describe the first aid measures which relatives can take.

● Force yourself to act quickly and decisively. Make persons who are excited or crying leave the immediate area of the patient.

● Call the physician immediately. Express your concern about a heart attack on the phone, but if possible do not allow the patient to overhear the diagnosis you suspect. Ask whether pain-killers, tranquilizers or heart drugs such as nitrates should be given to the patient.

● Allow the patient to decide whether to sit up or to lie down. Make sure that fresh air is available and help open articles of clothing which impede breathing, such as a tie, collar, jacket, bodice, brassiere, or belt.

● Take note of the pulse rate occasionally (the rate per minute, whether it is regular or irregular) because this information is important for the physician when he arrives.

● Your most important duty, however, is to remain with the patient. You may alleviate the mortal dread common in this situation by offering sympathy and fulfilling the desire to feel the closeness of another human being. Hold and stroke the hand, calm and console the patient while remaining outwardly calm yourself.

Immediate help through medication

The patient often reaches for nitrates in order to relieve the unbearable pain. There is nothing wrong with taking nitrates even though the intense pain of an acute heart attack can usually not be relieved by them. Other drugs (such as digitalis) should not be taken without the physician's order. The doctor will attempt to calm down the patient with drugs, usually administered intravenously, and to relieve pain. You should request that the physician accompany the patient to the hospital in order to be able to counter any complications, unless an ambulance is equipped with trained paramedical personnel. Moreover, you should give the patient a list of the drugs being taken, as well as your phone number.

Give clear directions to the driver

When you call the emergency number for an ambulance and a physician, you should keep in mind that the information you give should be very concise and precise:
- Who is the patient and who is calling?
- What happened?
- Where did it happen (in which part of the city, at which street, intersection, in which part of the house, on which floor, and what is the telephone number)?

It often happens that valuable time is lost searching for the location of the patient. The author spent many years working with such emergency cases and suggests the following action:
- Ask someone to wave to the ambulance with a noticeable object, at night with a flashlight, in order to attract the driver's attention.
- Leave the door of the apartment or house open.
- Block the elevator on the ground floor by holding the door open.
- Turn on the lights to illuminate the house number or the entire apartment.
- Also we hope that soon all persons will be familiar with the emergency telephone number.

What Should the Patient and Relatives NOT Do?

You should not wait under any circumstances, nor delay in taking action. You must realize that 60% of all deaths caused by heart attack occur within the first few hours of the symptoms, so you should act immediately and not allow valuable time to pass without a physician's supervision. Your time of decision-making should be as short as possible.

Life-endangering arrhythmias can occur abruptly, and can be successfully treated only in a hospital. It is necessary to overcome the understandable, but futile, hope that the symptoms will disappear by themselves. Also, the desire to stay at home to avoid hospitalization and its discomforts must be suppressed. You should not take any risks, especially if you have information that the patient has sustained a previous heart attack and that this episode is a re-infarction. We cannot repeat too often that it is imperative to go directly to the hospital when a heart attack is suspected.

Do not waste time if a heart attack is suspected

Immediate Measures for Resuscitation

The worst that can happen, either at home or on the road, is a cardiac arrest which is caused by the abnormal heart rhythm in the early phase. As a consequence, the heart can no longer pump blood to the vital organs of the body, resulting in a severe lack of oxygen. The brain is the most exposed to this danger because irreversible damage can be prevented only in the first three minutes. In such a case, artificial respiration and heart massage may save the patient's life.

The body in need of oxygen

All other complications, such as cardiac insufficiency, which may arise after a heart attack and which may cause death, usually cannot be recognized or alleviated by the layman. However, these complications usually arise at a later time when medical assistance is already available.

How to recognize cardiac arrest

It is not difficult to recognize cardiac arrest because the patients' condition changes rapidly. They become unconscious and their face or hands turn a blue-gray color. They may gasp for air

59

or make a snoring sound, or their pulse and breathing may not be perceptible at all. This situation poses a clear danger to life, but if you take immediate and appropriate measures, you may still save it. By means of artificial respiration and strong, effective heart massage, it is possible to revive breathing and the circulation to supply the heart, brain and kidneys with oxygen until the physician arrives on the scene or the patient arrives at the hospital.

Heart massage and artificial respiration (mouth-to-mouth or mouth-to-nose)

How to save a life
1. Place the patient immediately flat on his back on a hard floor.
2. With your closed fist or the edge of your hand hit the breastbone. Rapidly check to see whether the heart is beating again by placing your ear on his chest or your finger on the main artery at the lateral aspect of the neck.

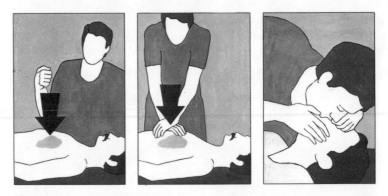

Resuscitation. These three pictures show the most important actions to be taken. *Left,* hitting the heart area. *Center,* heart massage. *Right,* mouth-to-mouth artificial respiration.

3. If the heart has not resumed beating, place one closed fist on the lower third of the breastbone, but not on the stomach, and the other closed fist on the upper third of the breastbone. Using your body weight and keeping your elbows straight, apply pressure to the breastbone in line with the spine at a consistent rate of 60 to 80 times per minute. Be sure to measure the rate of this massage with a clock or watch that has a second hand.

4. After each fifth time of pushing on the breastbone, it is important to give artificial respiration, since heart massage without artificial respiration is of no value. Placing one hand on the forehead, the second one under the chin, push the lower jaw forward and against the upper jaw. Keep the mouth closed by pressing your thumb on it.

This can also be done with two persons

5. Place the patient's hands above and to the back of the head. Breathe deeply and place your mouth over the patient's nose. Blow air in for three seconds and then allow the patient to exhale for two seconds. The chest and the upper abdomen should expand when you blow air in. If you prefer to use the mouth-to-mouth method, pinch the patient's nose shut. Then repeat the heart massage as described in the third paragraph. In this five-to-one ratio of five massaging motions to one artificial breath for the patient, continue the process without pause.

You have only 3 minutes!

Those who have practiced this method (as in a first-aid course) will be able to apply it in the case of an emergency. However, you must act immediately and should not waste time in long telephone conversations or in any other way. You should keep in mind that you have only three minutes to restore life-sustaining circulation.

Since heart massage and artificial respiration can be very tiring, it may be better for two persons to cooperate. However, someone who seriously attempts to overcome the crucial period until the physician arrives or the patient reaches the hospital, often forgets his own fatigue. In such situations in which there is nothing to lose and everything to gain, the normal reaction is to continue tirelessly.

5. What Happens in the Intensive Care Unit?

Life-Saving Intensive Care

When the patient arrives at the hospital, the physician on duty must first of all either confirm or eliminate the diagnosis of heart attack by listening to the symptoms, what measures have already been taken, and the circumstances surrounding the attack. The spouse of the patient should not forget the list of drugs which have been taken. The EKG is taken immediately and sometimes indicates certain changes, but may not indicate anything unusual in the early stage. In these cases, the changes become evident in the EKG only a few hours or even a few days later.

Confirming a heart attack

Blood tests may yield more information in most cases. It is possible to measure the amount of certain enzymes which the damaged heart muscle releases into the blood stream. Since these enzymes indicate the time and course of the response to the heart attack, they must be checked daily.

If a heart attack can be ruled out as a possibility, by a normal EKG and enzyme level, then the patient is transferred to a general ward. A few days of observation should reveal the cause of the symptoms which resulted in the emergency. In some cases an impending heart attack is discovered, which would have occurred sooner or later if the necessary steps are not taken. In other cases, the cause of the pain has little to do with the heart, but instead originates in the spinal column (see page 37) or in an emotional or nervous disorder.

If a heart attack is indicated or suspected, the patient is transferred as soon as possible to the intensive care unit. It is understandable that relatives and the patient himself often view this admission with mixed feelings.

Heinz P., a sixty-year-old railroad official remembers: "I sustained a heart attack while I was in Munich visiting my children. The fire department rushed me to the nearest hospital where the physician on duty took an EKG. The immediate diagnosis was that I had sustained a minor heart attack and that it would be best if I were admitted to the intensive care unit where I could be observed and treated more effectively. My wife was relieved, but I began to worry. Although the nurses and physicians took good care of me, I simply could not grow accustomed to the strict order to stay in bed, the constant coming and goings of the staff, the restless woman in the bed next to mine, or to the urinary catheter."

Is the discomfort experienced by this patient in the intensive care unit absolutely necessary? As a matter of fact it is necessary and his wife was right to be relieved when he was admitted to the unit. It is only natural that he did not like to lie in a horizontal position for three days. Regulation of the bowel movement and urination may prevent disturbances of the heart rhythm. Unfortunately the restlessness of the other patients does distract the patient and a death in the hospital might depress him even further.

However, all these disadvantages are far out-weighed by excellent treatment offered at such intensive care units, which is not found in general medical wards. Since the first days following the heart attack are the most crucial ones, the therapy and observation of the patient must be constant. The patient is usually monitored by an instrument which detects any irregularities in the cardiac rhythm.

At the same time a device is inserted into the vein of the arm or of the collar bone region, by means of which necessary drugs to relieve pain or to calm the patient can be infused over a period of several days. Moreover, the inner pressure of the major vein leading to the heart can be measured.

The recovery from an acute heart attack may be severely impaired by irregularities in the cardiac rhythm and by circulatory complications. Irregularities of the cardiac rhythm which cause the heart rate to either increase or decrease must be treated immediately by infusions of necessary medication, because a decrease in the pumping activity of the heart would result in an insufficient oxygen supply to the brain. This dangerous situation can only be prevented by the use of a pacemaker in certain circumstances.

Various technical means are available to make the use of a pacemaker possible. The pacemaker relies on the principle that an electrical impulse can stimulate the heart to beat regularly. This impulse is generated by a battery and reaches the heart through a wire passed into a vein. In most cases, the pacemaker can be removed after a few days when the regulatory system of the heart regains its normal functioning (also see page 75).

Any weakness of the heart or other circulatory problems must also be monitored constantly. It is possible to increase the pumping action, strengthen the heart, and improve kidney function and fluid output, raise or lower the blood pressure by means of drug therapy. It is hoped that the consequences of a heart attack can be controlled in this manner, in addition to a supply of oxygen through the nose.

During the crucial stage after the heart attack, the intensive care unit offers a maximum of security with the best technical equipment and highly skilled personnel; although certain discomforts and great financial burden to the family are unavoidable. Visiting hours are arranged as conveniently as possible, but children and flowers cannot be allowed. Moreover, there is very little space for the personal belongings of the patient. Since nurses and physicians are in attendance around the clock, they are available for consultation at any time. The relatives and the patient should take advantage of this situation in order to gain information which may help the patient overcome the fears of the first few days after the heart attack. This psychological consideration is important for the patient and the relatives.

Young patients in particular experience emotional distress when they become conscious of having just escaped death. The patient's previous feeling of well-being and security is undermined. Although the advantage of the intensive care unit is its sophisticated equipment, it is the sight of all that machinery which often causes fear and insecurity in the patient. Yet such fear could

be allayed in a sympathetic and honest discussion with the physician. Such conversations can play an important role during the early phase of recovery.

The spouse and the patient will often avoid talking with the physician about the condition, because they may think the physician too busy or be afraid they will not understand his explanation. Since they are also afraid of depressing or frightening news, some of the much-needed discussion with physicians may never take place.

Let your loved ones share your feelings

It is still more problematic, however, when the spouse and the patient avoid any serious conversation and engage in meaningless chatter about the weather or the food. Although each does not want to upset the other, each may actually feel lonelier by avoiding important topics. Even though it is natural to avoid serious conversation in the first few days when the patient is gravely ill and under sedation, it is not acceptable if serious talk is avoided for several weeks. The patient may repress fears, making it more difficult to overcome them. Later, the patient may minimize or overcompensate for the early stage of recovery, instead of trying immediately to start for a new life together with loved ones. If the spouse tries to protect the patient from the truth by making light conversation, avoiding topics such as the children's education, the financial situation or the business, this may deprive the patient of the opportunity to participate and make decisions as was true earlier. Instead, husband and wife should cooperate in resolving the problems which arise. Only by offering advice while the patient is ill, can one help him or her to regain confidence. Whether you are a patient or are visiting a patient, you should engage in open and frank, intimate conversation rather than idle chatter. By sharing your feelings and empathizing with the other person, both of you will gain from the experience.

Early Mobilization

Ten or twenty years ago, heart attack patients suffered not only from the intense pain, the threat to life, and forced early retirement, but also from rigid confinement to bed because it was believed that the heart muscle scar tissue would require at least six weeks to heal. Often patients who were intent on moving around a little could do so only at night when they felt that they were not being observed. However, later studies revealed that prolonged confinement to bed causes not only psychological, but physical problems, as for example the increased tendency to coagulation and thrombo-embolism, impaired circulation and a

Disadvantages of prolonged confinement to bed

65

tendency to develop pneumonia. Cardiologists in the 1960's became less strict about bed rest and began to encourage early mobilization when they saw that this caused no complications. In 1968 the World Health Organization reviewed these studies and recommended early mobilization as standard practice.

Since then most hospitals practice early mobilization if no contra-indications are present. The patient usually rests in bed or a chair for several days and then gradually increases activities. Already in the intensive care unit a nurse or a physical therapist begins working with the patient twice each day if this is feasible. The therapist begins with breathing and relaxation exercises and then, while carefully observing the pulse and respiration rate, proceeds to active and passive exercise of muscles in the arms and legs.

Getting up again

The immediate goals of washing oneself (while sitting in bed) and the use of a commode should be attained within a few days. After exercising larger sets of muscles while lying down and sitting on the bed for several days, the patient may stand up and walk around the room, eat at the table with his legs wrapped up and go to the bathroom by himself. Eventually the patient will be able to walk a little further, perform more exercises while sitting, and mount stairs slowly. He should be observed by means of a Holter monitor which he straps to himself. Before climbing stairs, the patient's ability to endure physical exertion may be tested by a bicycle ergometer examination (see page 42). Then the gymnastic

Climbing stairs and walking

exercises, climbing of stairs and walking can be increased gradually so that the younger patients may participate in a coronary gymnastic group before leaving the hospital. Older patients or those who have sustained a more severe or complicated heart attack may not be able to increase their exercises so quickly, and may have to stay in the hospital for a longer period.

Cooperation between the attending physician, the nurse, or the physical therapist and the patient plays an important role in the early mobilization, as does the close observation and discussion of complications, irregularities in the cardiac rhythm, and changes in the pulse rate.

Other advantages of early mobilization

The advantages of early mobilization lie in the prevention of impaired coagulation with thromboses and embolisms, as well as of pneumonia. Improved blood circulation and heart muscle function also appear. The patient recovers more quickly in the psychological aspect when able to move about freely without

66

Plan for Mobilization

This step-by-step mobilization plan for the physical therapy of heart attack patients must be adapted to suit each individual case.

Step 1

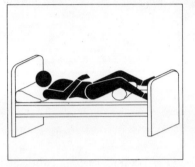

In bed (intensive care unit): passive exercises, relaxation exercises. Immediate goal: assuagement of fear.

Step 2

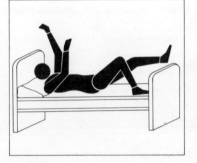

In bed: active exercises for the small, then larger sets of muscles. Intermittently: relaxing breathing exercises. Sitting up slightly with head and knees supported. Immediate goal: ability to wash oneself in bed with back support, use of commode with help of nurse (legs should be wrapped or support stockings used). Future goal: calmness, relaxation, improved blood circulation of the heart.

Step 3

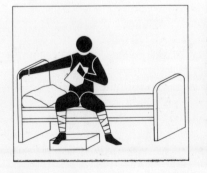

Rhythmic exercises of the large sets of muscles while lying down and on the side. Stabilizing exercises while sitting at the side of the bed, legs wrapped. Exercises involving the feet. Immediate goal: being able to read, eat, and wash while sitting at the edge of the bed, sitting in a chair, legs wrapped, and using a foot stool. Future goal: relaxation, calmness, improved blood circulation of the heart.

Step 1

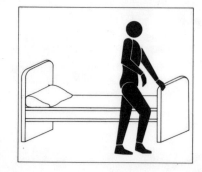

Increasing previous exercises. Standing at the foot of the bed for a short period of time. Walking in the room. Immediate goal: washing at basin while sitting and going to the bathroom alone. Future goal: relaxation, calmness, improved blood circulation of the heart.

Step 2

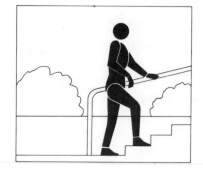

Coordination exercises, and possibly sitting exercises. Walking on flat surface, then stairs (stop and check pulse). Ergometry twenty-five to fifty watts. Immediate goal: walking in the house and eventually in the garden. Future goal: relaxation, calmness, improved blood circulation in the heart.

Step 3

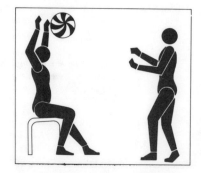

Stabilization of ability to exercise in a gymnasium. If possible, group therapy with several coronary patients, and eventually ergometric training (pulse control, rest) without pushing or forced breathing. Ergometry fifty to seventy-five watts.

direct supervision. The patient may also develop a better relationship with the physician when not confined to bed for six weeks as previous practice had dictated. In those hospitals where a physical therapist is not readily available, the patient should request a list of exercises to perform alone during the day.

6. What Is the Emotional Reaction to a Heart Attack?

Fear and Depression

When we discussed this topic with our patients and our publishers in order to make sure that it could be understood by laypersons, the publishers were struck by the manner in which coronary patients concealed their fears. The patients often do not concede to their physician or themselves that they fear for their lives. But since all patients probably harbor such fears, we must all learn how to overcome them.

Learning to deal with fear

In some patients fear leads to depression which must be treated. For a short period of time, anti-depressant drugs may be taken without side-effects, but this is the physician's decision.

It is also possible that patients suffer from another type of depression, the symptoms of which are physical rather than emotional. It may also be helpful if patients talk about these fears and depression with their spouses in order to confront and thus overcome these problems more quickly.

Repression and Dissimulation

Whereas some patients are hypochondriacs and exaggerate or invent symptoms, coronary patients often dissimulate their symptoms and their fears of developing life-threatening complications. The manner in which a coronary patient describes symptoms often gives the cardiologist an indication about his or her psychological state. Whereas the coronary patient tends to minimize his disease and insist that nothing is really wrong, the neurotic heart patient draws attention to complaints by dramatic descriptions.

The non-medical wife of a professor of medicine who is a friend of ours made the diagnosis "heart attack," but the professor angrily denied this, saying that he simply had something lodged in his esophagus or wind pipe. Similarly, a radiologist recalls that he suspected a heart attack in his own case, but had attempted to mislead his physician by describing different symptoms in order to avoid facing the truth.

Extremely ambitious persons who are very active in their careers often react in a manner involving both repression and dissimulation by insisting that everything is well again and that they are ready to take up all their former activities.

Advice for the family   We hope that by drawing attention to these typical and possibly hazardous psychological reactions to a myocardial infarction, we can warn and be of help not only to patients, but also to relatives.

We also hope that the thoughts communicated in this section will encourage an open discussion with the physician. In our experience with heart attack patients we have found that the fears repressed in the first few weeks often turn into aggression. Many patients learn to realize and finally accept their situation with its limitations and possibilities only toward the end of their stay in the hospital.

How Should One React?

How should one change one's attitude in order to adjust more easily to the consequences of a heart attack?

It must be emphasized that it is impossible to generalize about reactions to a heart attack. Obviously the reaction of someone who tends to repress and dissimulate reality is certainly quite different from the reaction of someone who tends to withdraw into a depression from which there appears to be no escape.

A narrow escape from death causes fear in everyone, although some persons are able to conceal it from others and sometimes even from themselves. In the days and weeks which pass after a heart attack, all patients at some time wonder about the meaning of their past and future life. At some point either in the intensive care unit, the rehabilitation center or at home, every patient goes through a phase in which the fear of death becomes a fear of life.

How shall life continue?

The crucial question then becomes: "How shall it continue?"

In our experience, patients who confront this question directly and make no attempt to evade it are likely to begin a new, happy life after the heart attack. They must summon all their courage to successfully overcome this phase of reflection and loneliness which has been called the 'journey through the desert' by more religious patients. A heart attack is not simply a minor mishap, but is instead a major event in the life of the patient and has great bearing on the remainder of his or her life. Moreover, as a Dutch cardiologist once said, there are more problems to be resolved in the patient's mind than in his heart. We therefore hope that your physician will also be a trusted companion who will be able to help you in overcoming this experience.

Family doctor as partner and helper

Such a physician plays an even more important, but also a more difficult role when surgery is required. Anyone who may need surgery is likely to see it only as a threat at first and will view it with fear, or at the very least, with mixed feelings.

7. Surgical Help

Heart surgery has undergone many important developments in the past ten years. As in all medical progress these developments may be overestimated by those who expect all problems to be immediately resolved, and who may not be aware of the limitations imposed on the rate of progress. But the developments are also underestimated by those who are sceptical of any progress and who view advances with apprehension. It seems necessary to us to introduce this chapter with such an observation, because we can understand why patients today seek the opinion of different experts in order to avoid either one of the two extremes. Also we *Surgery is not* would like to emphasize that surgical intervention is only one part *a cure-all* of the recovery process and that its success is dependent on a fully integrated program of rehabilitation. Therefore the patient who thinks he can avoid making necessary changes in life-style solely by means of surgical intervention will be very disappointed.

What exactly is a by-pass operation and an aneurysmectomy? When is such surgery indicated?

The By-Pass Operation

The by-pass In a by-pass operation those parts of the coronary vessels which have been blocked through changes in the vessel walls are literally by-passed. Part of a vessel is used to connect the aorta to a point beyond the occlusion in the coronary vessel. The vessel with which the by-pass is constructed can be taken from a vein in the leg or an artery in the chest cavity. In the course of the operation a number of such by-passes may be constructed. The operation is most likely to be successful if there are two, three, or more occlusions in the coronary vessels which are localized and clearly

73

demarcated, and if the muscles of the ventricle still function properly.

Ventriculography and coronary angiography have become more and more important because only these diagnostic procedures can determine whether conditions are suitable for surgery or whether long-term drug therapy should be favored. A more detailed description of this operation would be beyond the scope of this book, but your cardiologist will certainly be able to inform you

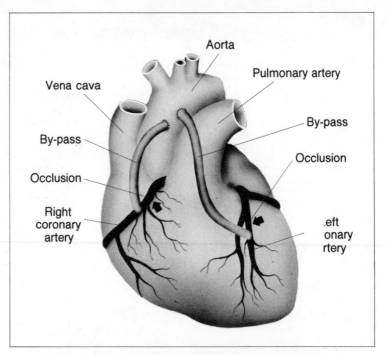

By-pass. Occlusions of two coronary arteries are by-passed. As a result of the by-pass, the blood from the aorta flows around the blockages into the coronary arteries.

about the procedure and can also suggest its possible advantages and disadvantages for you as an individual patient. Again we would like to emphasize that the success of a by-pass operation depends largely on the rehabilitation preceding and following it.

Aneurysmectomy

An aneurysm is a localized sac-like bulge in the heart-muscle (or in a large vessel) which develops as a result of certain changes in the connective tissue (for example after a heart attack, see p. 46). The different stages of such aneurysms can be determined by ventriculography and coronary angiography. Only extensive aneurysms must be operated upon, especially if they result in irregular cardiac rhythm or congestive heart failure when they cannot be controlled by drug-therapy. Often a by-pass operation and an aneurysmectomy are performed at the same time.

Other Blood Vessel Surgery

Today it is also feasible to replace blocked vessels in other parts of the body with artificial vessels. Such operations are performed in the arteries of the legs, in the pelvic area, for example, in the aortic fork where occlusions appear to be enhanced by smoking, or in certain areas of the neck and brain where changes could lead to a stroke. It seems particularly important to us to mention this type of surgery in this context because more than half of the coronary patients also suffer from occlusions of varying degrees in the legs or the pelvic area. However, these occlusions are rarely so serious as to require surgery.

The Pacemaker

Alfred N., who is 64 years old, sustained a heart attack on New Year's Eve. He would never have believed this diagnosis if it had not been confirmed in the intensive care unit, because he never experienced any feeling of pressure or tightness, any shortness of breath or any other symptom which would have made him aware of heart problems. Shortly before midnight he had felt nauseous, weak, tired, and dizzy, and had perspired profusely. Later his wife stated that she had felt as if he had been on the verge of fainting before the ambulance arrived. Since she had taught physical education, she knew how to measure the pulse and was shocked when she could barely count 40 beats per minute. She again checked the pulse rate, but her husband's pulse was frighteningly slow.

Her observation was confirmed in the hospital where they were also informed that he would need a temporary pacemaker. As a result of the heart attack, a certain area of the heart muscle, which had played an important role in regulating the heart beat, had been damaged. They were told that this area which is part of the conduction system of the heart and plays an important role in automatic heart action could possibly recover within a few days

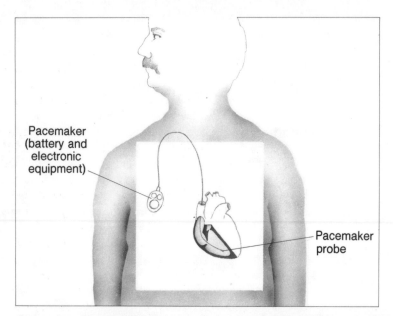

Pacemaker. The small pacemaker (battery and electronic equipment) is implanted under the skin in the chest. The probe goes through a vein into the right heart chamber.

Restoring proper heart rate artificially

but that in the meantime the heart rate would have to be controlled by artificial means. As soon as the heart rate falls below 30 beats per minute, the blood supply to the body, in particular to the brain, is insufficient and may result in cramps and loss of consciousness.

There was no time for deliberations or objections. The area

76

under the left collar bone was locally anesthetized, the skin was separated, and the probe of the pacemaker was pushed toward the heart through a large vein. The procedure was carried out with the help of x-rays. The other end of the probe was connected to the pacemaker which was placed in a small box and taped to the upper arm. The patient's condition improved dramatically with the pulse having been restored to 70 beats per minute.

In many cases the rhythmic center and the conduction system of the heart recover within a few days so that the probe of the pacemaker may be removed painlessly from the right ventricle. If this is not the case, then the pacemaker must be permanently implanted in order to normalize the heart rate.

Implantation of a pacemaker

The pacemaker is implanted through a minor surgical intervention which involves only a local anesthetic. Through a small cut in the skin of the shoulder-neck area a thin wire with the probe of the pacemaker is inserted in a large vein and pushed toward the heart. The pacemaker is attached to the other end of the probe and is implanted under the skin. The pacemaker consists of a material compatible with the body in which the source of energy, a battery and other minute electronic parts, are contained. The incisions in the skin heal within a few days and then the stitches can be removed.

The implanted pacemaker has sufficient energy to last for a few years after which it must be renewed by means of a minor procedure. Modern lithium pacemakers are particularly advantageous because they last longer, are small, and weigh only 3½ ounces.

The demand pacemaker

Most patients today wear a demand pacemaker which supplies electrical impulses automatically only when an electronic detector attached to the same wire determines that the heart rate falls below the normal 70 beats per minute. Although these technical devices are generally dependable, the patient must become accustomed to checking the functioning of the pacemaker once or twice daily by taking his pulse. Usually problems with the pacemaker are rare during the first few weeks after implantation.

Problems with the pacemaker

If, however, there should be a problem with the heart rate, it may be caused either by the heart itself, the connecting wire, or the pacemaker, for example, if the batteries are weak. The physician who implanted the pacemaker should be able to determine the cause of any problems and should check it regularly. If the pulse does not fall below 45 beats per minute, the patient may wait a day or two to see the doctor. If any of the following symptoms

77

appear, the patient should also notify his physician and relate any major changes in pulse:
- Shortness of breath, dizziness, short periods of numbness or unconsciousness;
- Prolonged fatigue or weakness;
- Swelling in legs, ankles, wrists, or arms;
- Discomfort in the chest or continued hiccups;
- Changes in the skin above the pacemaker.

Preventing damage resulting from pressure

The patient should have few additional complaints and should take care only to avoid putting pressure on the implant with articles of clothing, bags, musical instruments, or sports equipment. Pressure on the implant could cause infection or a rupture which may be recognized by redness, pain, fluid formation, swelling, or changes in the skin. If the pacemaker is implanted in the skin of the abdomen the patient should wear suspenders instead of belts.

The patient will be informed by those who were involved in the implantation how often a return for follow-up care is necessary and after how many years the pacemaker should be exchanged for a new one. The patient should make the first appointment for a check-up immediately after having the pacemaker implanted. Instead of taking his pulse himself daily, the patient may buy one of the instruments available to control pacemakers, but these are rather expensive.

As soon as the heart attack and the small scar from the implantation of the pacemaker are well-healed, the patient will probably wish to take short trips. He or she should never forget to take his pacemaker identification along, which should always be kept with other personal papers.

The final question which we will discuss is whether other magnetic fields such as those from an electric shaver or an electric motor have any influence on the pacemaker.

In general, electrical instruments and metal detectors used in airports do not cause any disturbances in pacemakers. Caution must be exercised only when the patient is in close contact with electric transformers, radar stations, electric arc-welders, microwave ovens or defective instruments. If the patient should suddenly feel numb, he should simply move away from the instrument. The pacemaker will then resume its normal activity.

Returning to normal life

Basically patients should be able to lead normal lives with the pacemaker. They may begin driving again since fitness to drive

Driving with
a pacemaker

should be the same as that of any other person. Seat belts should not cause any problems with the pacemaker or the wire and no complaints have been reported, although it is conceivable that in an accident the seat belt across the shoulder could cause the pacemaker to malfunction. But this would probably happen only if the patient is sitting in the right front seat and had the pacemaker implanted on the right side rather than in the left side, as is commonly done. Patients who would like to avoid this minor risk could simply sit in the back. Patients may travel by bus, plane, train, boat, or cable car, and they may bathe, shower, swim, or use the sauna at will. They may perform any of the usual activities characteristic of their age, including physical and sexual activities. It would be absolutely wrong and a shame if patients did not make the most of life with the pacemaker. Certain small inconveniences are unavoidable, but in general it should be possible to enjoy life again.

8. Comprehensive Follow-Up Care

Goals and Means of Rehabilitation

The term 'treatment and therapy' is known by all to incorporate every measure which helps eliminate or reduce the symptoms of disease (for example, pain). The term 'rehabilitation' is more difficult to define and is disputed among physicians. Some use rehabilitation to designate only a certain treatment method, for example, exercise therapy, while others use it to designate pension and insurance plans which cover the patient when he leaves the hospital. However, the goals of rehabilitation are much broader.

What we mean by rehabilitation

First of all, rehabilitation denotes the compensation for irreversible damage through other functions of the organism which are still possible. The classic example of such compensation is the person who has had a leg amputated yet becomes an excellent skier, better in fact than healthy persons because he compensates or even overcompensates for the loss of his limb. Heart attack patients may compensate in a similar manner.

Secondly, rehabilitation also denotes secondary prevention. It means preventing progress of a chronic disease, coronary heart disease. Thirdly, rehabilitation denotes full restoration of the patients' life-time activities so that they may be able to contribute to progress and society.

Improved life-expectan- cy

Thus the goal of rehabilitation is not simply to prolong the life of the patient, but to improve its quality. Rehabilitation encompasses not only the physical well-being but also the return of the patient to occupation and social circle (friends, family, marriage.) The goal of longevity combined with the best possible life can be expressed as, "not only to bring more years to life, but also to bring more life into the years."

After many years of experience in hospitals we are certain that this ambitious goal can be undertaken successfully if the patient

80

and physician cooperate, beginning in the intensive care unit. Rehabilitation must also be as comprehensive as possible to include not only the prescription of drugs, but also diet, physical activity, overcoming of fear and depression, as well as counseling on the return to work.

Arguments in Favor of Clinical Early Rehabilitation (in Europe)

The ambitious goals described may be met at home under the supervision of the personal physician if no complications arise from the heart attack and the patient and physician are able to cooperate. But how often are the conditions so favorable? May we suggest that home care be preceded by a structured program of rehabilitation in a special center or clinic for rehabilitation? We are discussing, of course, the present situation in Germany for patients after a myocardial infarction, a situation which may sound almost utopian to the American reader.

t is easier
with a group

The difficult process of becoming accustomed to a new life-style is made easier in a place where group therapy is possible. In such a center, the patient can be informed and encouraged to adopt the life-style appropriate for the rest of his life. As a participant in a controlled group, the patient is motivated more easily. In discussion groups, the patient is made aware of his personal risk factors and can then reduce them, for example, by attending non-smoking sessions.

What are the important goals of a rehabilitation program after the discharge from the hospital?
• controlling the individual risk factors
• practicing the self-discipline necessary to comply with long-term drug therapy (see p. 86);
• maintaining the individualized exercise therapy.

The success of this program is of course also dependent on the cooperation of the family, in particular of the spouse.

In a later chapter we shall discuss the particular problems which the return of heart attack patients may pose for their marriages. They must avoid the two extremes of behavior, playing the role of a spoiled child as well as the totally helpless approach.

81

Outpatient Coronary Care
(Anti-Coronary Club)

*The new
life-style*

The adoption of a new life-style which promotes the health of the patient and involves regaining his confidence and putting his fears aside, is made easier for him if he can meet once or twice a week with other patients under the supervision of a physician. Many such groups and clubs have been founded successfully in every city and town with the cooperation of experienced and competent physicians.

*Cooperating
with an
experienced
physician*

Such a club for coronary patients does not involve formal or legal statutes, but instead is an informal gathering of twenty to twenty-five patients. A physician and physical therapist (a psychologist, dietician, and sociologist may also be present) supervise a one to two hour weekly program of physical activity to improve the blood circulation and general health of the patients. In one such group under our guidance, all patients are invited who live in that particular area and have the permission of their physician. In many groups patients are accepted, when they attain 75 watts on a bicycle ergometer and when high blood pressure, irregular cardiac rhythm and congestive heart failure are treated. The age of the group ranges from 35 to 70 years of age. While some patients had sustained only a minor heart attack, others suffered from various complications. After warming up, the group exercises together. Breathing and relaxation exercises are interspersed, and this part of the session ends with a game and a shower.

*Discussions
help*

A discussion follows about the elimination and reduction of risk factors, and about the problems a patient encounters after being discharged from the intensive care unit. Common experiences such as shock, fear and depression are overcome in an atmosphere of sympathy, mutual understanding, and encouragement. Patients often emphasize that all those who participate in the discussion groups feel better as soon as they can share their feelings and no longer feel as isolated as they did right after the heart attack. In the course of six to twelve months participants in this medically supervised group become independent and learn how to help themselves. Wives of those patients who do not join such groups relate how much more difficult it is for these patients to return to a normal life-style.

82

Spouses may also gain much from such groups when they see how the patients are able to return to a more normal life-style and learn how to deal with the patients on a personal basis.

Unfortunately, no complete lists of such groups are yet available, but perhaps your physician can put you into contact with one.

Insurance Company Involvement on Post-Myocardial Infarction Care and Rehabilitation in the United States

The national extent of insurance company reimbursement of cardiac rehabilitation programs is unknown. Various projects, however, are being conducted and closely observed regarding their cost-effectiveness. For example, one Blue Cross and Blue Shield Plan has embarked on a cooperative state-wide evaluation of cardiac rehabilitation with responsible members of the medical profession and heart association. In this program the rehabilitation team is comprised of a cardiologist, exercise physiologist, nutritionist and psychologist.

In many areas the Blue plans will not include reimbursement for either ergometric testing or exercise programs, limiting their coverage to the acute in-hospital phase only. This is done in an effort to hold down costs of health care, operating on the philosophy that insurance is for disease only, and not for rehabilitation or prevention, laudable as these may be. When the Blue plans refuse coverage, major medical coverage may fill the gap.

9. Learning to Live with the Effects of a Heart Attack

Different Interpretations of Coronary Symptoms after a Heart Attack

Patients who have sustained a heart attack naturally assume that any complaints in the heart area are related to their myocardial infarction. However, dyscardia and other complaints caused by different parts of the body (such as the vertebral column) can be projected onto the heart after the heart attack just as prior to it, even in healthy persons. Heart attack patients understandably become more sensitive to their heart with the good intention of taking better care of it. As a result, they tend to worry about minor pains which they would have barely noticed earlier. Many symptoms, completely unrelated to the heart, are then thought to be caused by it. Fortunately, this stage is of short duration in most cases because the more time passes after the heart attack, the more confidence the patient gains and the less concerned he becomes about minor pains. The patient should consult his physician if regaining his emotional balance takes longer. By means of exact descriptions and the self-testing methods explained on p. 34 the patient can learn to distinguish a true angina pectoris from a false one, dyscardia.

Regaining confidence

True angina may be reduced, be the same, or be more pronounced after a heart attack.

Mr. A.D., 50 years of age, came to our clinic one day riding his bike. He had sustained a heart attack 10 weeks earlier, but now was able to attain 100 watts on the bicycle ergometer and while walking. He has only one complaint which is that he still is made aware of his heart after meals, on cool mornings, after rapidly climbing stairs, when the weather changes, and when he is upset or under time pressure.

Being aware of one's heart

84

What usually happens after a heart attack? Will one continue to have heart problems? What can be done to prevent them? Angina pectoris, which occurs rarely, lasts only 2 to 5 minutes, and disappears when standing or sitting down and can be treated successfully with drugs such as nitrates and beta blockers. The nitrates should be taken in a dose sufficiently large to prevent attacks of angina pectoris. For quick relief in cases of emergency or unexpected increase in chest pain, ask your physician for a special pill rapidly absorbed from under the tongue or a spray. You should always take these nitrates along with you wherever you go. Moreover, you should ask what the maximum dose is in order to know how much of the drug you can take on a day when the pain is particularly severe.

Prevention with nitrates

What should you do if the chest pains do not become milder or less frequent, but instead increase in frequency, duration and intensity? What should you do if you suddenly feel pain after the slightest physical exertion? You are probably in a new phase of your coronary heart disease and you should immediately inform your physician about it. He must have a detailed description because he cannot know what you do not tell him. You should take your new symptoms seriously and act immediately to prevent re-infarction. We cannot emphasize this point strongly enough. An apathetic attitude characterized by the remark "what came up by itself, will disappear by itself" could have grave consequences for the patient. If the complaints are particularly frequent and severe, and cannot be controlled with the drugs discussed in the chapter on long-term drug therapy, then a coronary angiography must be performed. This examination will make it possible to decide whether a by-pass operation is necessary. Over 90% of those who are operated upon are free of symptoms after surgery.

Becoming Productive and Enjoying Life Again

Story of a former sports man

A typical example will demonstrate the importance of complying with drug therapy.

A 45-year-old down-hill skiier who had also been active in other kinds of sports (soccer and skiing instruction) developed coronary heart disease (he smoked and was overweight.) In the past two years he had given up his ski tours because of his angina pectoris and his growing fear of hurting himself. Only another avid skiier can understand what such a sacrifice actually means.

After a comprehensive program of rehabilitation including weight-loss, anti-smoking clinics, and long-term drug therapy, the patient again took up cross-country skiing and returned to the regular skiing slopes. Since he had a tendency to develop a high pulse rate as a result of exhaustion, he had received a prescription for beta blockers and had been advised to take nitrate tablets whenever he needed them. The patient had, however, misunderstood this advice.

*Misunder-
stood advice*

The patient was under the impression that he could take the tablets only after suffering an attack of angina pectoris which he could not overcome by "walking through" it. His ski trips were miserable until he became accustomed to taking the tablets 15 minutes prior to skiing. He now enjoys skiing as much as he had earlier.

This advice to prevent angina pectoris of course also applies to emotional stress and physical activities other than skiing which cause angina pectoris.

*Begin with a
smaller dose*

The patient had also developed headaches after taking a whole nitrate tablet (5mg). He was able to eliminate this side-effect by taking only half the tablet at a time, waiting 10 minutes to take the second half.

If we as physicians expect a high degree of compliance from the patient and in fact would like him to become a specialist in his particular disease, then we should provide him with the necessary information about long-term drug therapy.

Long-Term Drug Therapy

In this section we shall attempt to teach a short course in drug therapy for the patient who uses the drugs rather than for the physician who prescribes them.

*Taking
medication
regularly*

Studies have shown that only part of the patients to whom drugs have been prescribed actually take them. Only one in five hypertensive patients takes his medication regularly. Aside from the high cost of medication could one reason be that patients need to know more about the drug they use three times a day and why they should take it? However, these questions are difficult to answer without causing controversy among physicians and pharmaceutical companies.

Physicians are afraid for good reasons that too much information could cause fear and misunderstanding. Therefore, we would like to make a few preliminary comments. In this chapter only groups of drugs are discussed which are used in the long-term treatment of the chronic phase of coronary heart disease. Drugs for emergency treatment, for example in the acute stage of a heart attack, are not mentioned. Moreover, particularities of individual cases should be considered by the attending physician.

Your doctor will advise you in the details

Often the physician is asked impatiently how long the drug must be continued. The frequent answer to this question is that the patient will probably have to take it for the rest of his life. The reason for this is that the drugs described in this chapter do not simply cure one symptom which appears temporarily and should be suppressed for this short period of time. Instead, these drugs are more like a prothesis which takes over a function the body itself can no longer perform.

Long-term drug treatment

As we grow older we must learn to accept different protheses, whether they be glasses, false teeth, or artificial limbs.
● If we re-examine patients whose condition has improved greatly, we usually find that they have complied with long-term drug therapy.
● We shall discuss briefly only those questions which are frequently raised by patients. These key words should then lead to further discussions with the physician. We hope to emphasize that it is possible to achieve satisfactory treatment by using various drugs and that different names or doses of drugs do not always indicate different treatment methods. We emphasize this point only to allay possible fears.
● Unfortunately, few patients know the names of the drugs they are taking and can speak only of "small white and large yellow pills." Since the physician must have more precise information about the medication the patient is taking, you should retain the name, group, and effect of your drugs.

Write down the names of your drugs

Drug treatment for "coronary insufficiency"
In the advanced stage of coronary heart disease a shortness of

87

blood and oxygen is developed in the heart muscle which is called "coronary insufficiency." This condition may be chronic or acute, which is to say that, it can be worsened by emotional stress or physical exertion. In order to alleviate the insufficient blood and oxygen supply and the resulting chest tightness (angina pectoris), we recommend the two major groups, nitrates and beta blockers.

Nitrates

Nitroglycerin has been used successfully to treat angina pectoris for over 100 years. In the course of time, other nitrates from the same major group have also been shown to be effective in both clinical and experimental tests. Thus their range of application could be broadened. Nitrates reduce the work load of the heart by widening the blood vessels and decreasing the peripheral resistance of the musculature. For this reason, nitrates are used not only to treat symptoms of heart pain and chest tightness, but also to treat the acute stages of impending heart attack as well as many forms of congestive heart failure.

Answering frequent questions

The following questions about nitrates are frequently raised:

Should strong drugs such as those in the nitrate group be used sparingly?
The answer is no, because the side-effects even of long-term drug therapy are harmless. These unusually effective and safe drugs which protect the heart and contribute to its functioning should be used generously as directed.

Should nitrates be taken only in the case of an attack of angina pectoris?
The answer is no, because nitrates should be taken preventively in situations which usually cause an attack of angina pectoris. In our opinion, nitrates are not taken as frequently as they should. All medications which contain isosorbitdinitrate are effective for approximately 4 hours, and should therefore be taken four to six times a day. (Be sure to read the package inserts with your drugs.) Since nitrates improve the function of the heart, they should be taken before, rather than after the symptoms of impaired blood circulation in the heart appear.

Should nitrates be taken even if they cause headaches?
The development of headaches depends on the individual's

tolerance for nitrates and also on the dosage prescribed. They will usually disappear after a certain period of time. Moreover, the headaches indicate that the nitrates are effectively widening the blood vessels of the head. The headaches may be reduced by taking the nitrates in lower doses, for example by taking half a tablet at a time.

Is it possible to become addicted to nitrates so that they lose their effectiveness in case of an emergency?
This fear has no basis, because patients addicted to nitroglycerin can overcome this habituation by refraining from the drug for two days. If the nitro capsules lose their effectiveness, it may be because the package is old. In the event that coronary heart disease should continue to progress, a higher dosage may be required.

Whereas patients taking other drugs such as beta blockers and digitalis must adhere to a strict daily dosage, those taking nitrates are allowed greater freedom. The patient should therefore know not only what the daily dosage is, but also what the maximum dosage is for a day when the pain is particularly strong. Needless to say, the patient should always have a reserve supply of nitrates on hand.

Beta blockers.
This group of drugs which has been in use only for a few years decreases the activity of the sympathetic nervous system. These drugs decrease the oxygen demand of the heart muscle and also lower the blood pressure and pulse rate. Irregularities of the cardiac rhythm as well as fear and restlessness can also be controlled. Since beta blockers have been shown to effectively complement nitrates, the two drugs are often prescribed in combination for long-term treatment. However, the combination
Undesirable side-effects does not produce side-effects except in the well-known case of contra-indications. Such contra-indications include bronchial asthma, a low pulse rate, chronically low blood pressure, rhythm disturbances, congestive heart failure, juvenile diabetes which has been difficult to control, and peripheral atherosclerosis.

Drugs to minimize irregularities in the cardiac rhythm
Not all irregularities of the cardiac rhythm are in need of

treatment. Treatment is indicated:

When treatment is necessary

- when the irregularities of cardiac rhythm impair the function of the heart (for example, a pulse which is too slow or too fast for the age of the patient);
- when the irregularities pose a threat to the life of the patient (for example bursts of premature ventricular beats);
- when the irregularities do not pose a threat but are very uncomfortable to the patient.

In such cases the disciplined intake of medication can play an important role. By *disciplined* we mean taking the exact amount prescribed at the correct time. Such discipline is important because the drugs are effective only for a certain period of time (for example, 8 hours) and must therefore be taken after a specific time period to ensure the maintenance of a sufficient blood concentration.

Digitalis

Assisting the contractions

Congestive heart failure may be caused not only by infectious disease (valve defects and myocarditis) or chronic hypertension, but also by coronary heart disease. In such cases the contractions of the heart muscle must be supported. However, only those heart muscles which work insufficiently require digitalis (which was originally made from foxglove). Digitalis allows the heart muscle to work more efficiently. The heart muscle cells require less oxygen and the heart can beat at a reduced and therefore more economical rate. Since digitalis is not habit forming, it may be taken for periods of years. In chronic congestive heart failure, the three "D's", a salt-free diet, digitalis, and diuretics, must be observed carefully in order to sustain life.

Anticoagulant drugs

The medical layman must be made aware of the controversial medical opinions on anticoagulant drugs in long-term drug therapy for prevention of heart attacks and re-infarctions. We would like to emphasize this point because the patient will probably be confronted with conflicting advice in the course of his

Are anticoagu-lants useful?

treatment. The patient will then begin to worry and because of this controversy not a single question about medication is posed as frequently as those concerning anticoagulant medications.

90

Anticoagulant drugs impede the formation of blood clots, but do not thin the blood, as is sometimes incorrectly assumed.

Many factors are involved in the progression of coronary heart disease. Since the formation of blood clots is a significant factor in this progression, anticoagulant drugs play an important role.

*Lowering the
risk of clot
formation*

Anticoagulant drugs per se cannot prevent a heart attack because the formation of blood clots is only one factor among many which causes heart attacks. The anticoagulant drugs can only lower the risk of suddenly blocking a coronary vessel with a blood clot.

Have medical studies shown that anticoagulant drugs are effective in the treatment of heart attack patients? Numerous studies have proven that patients treated correctly with anticoagulant drugs are less threatened by re-infarction than those who are not treated with these drugs. Additional studies have also demonstrated that the survival rate among patients treated with anticoagulant drugs is higher than among those not treated with them.

However, other studies have shown that anticoagulant drugs do not play a significant role in the long-term treatment to prevent re-infarction. Such conflicting conclusions may be due either to inaccurate control of the "Quick" prothrombin time levels or to the fact that the number of patients examined was too small to ensure unambiguous results.

There is also disagreement over how long anticoagulants may be taken. Although it has been generally agreed that anticoagulants are effective for 2 to 3 years after a heart attack, their continued effectiveness is disputed.

The following points of advice are important for anyone taking anticoagulants:

*Important
advice*

1. Always carry your Quick levels (prothrombin time) with you. The desirable Quick's values lie between 10 and 25%, or about twice the control time.
2. Have the Quick's test repeated as prescribed and keep a record of the values.
3. Take your medication regularly in the prescribed dosage.
4. Do not take additional medication for pain, rheumatism, or colds (particularly aspirin) without the permission of your physician, because even non-prescription drugs can have a harmful effect on the coagulation of blood.

5. Inform every physician and dentist you visit that you are taking anticoagulants. You should not receive intramuscular injections.
6. Pay attention to any tendency toward bleeding and to the following warning signs: blue marks on your skin; bleeding of nose and gums; brownish discoloration or blood in the urine; and bright red blood in the bowel movement or tarry stools. In these instances stop taking the medication and contact your physician for instructions.
7. If you have a bleeding wound or injury press a sterile compress or clean towel on it until the bleeding stops or the doctor can be reached.

Patients who cannot be treated with anticoagulants for various reasons such as age or peptic ulcers, may be treated instead with certain other drugs which prevent the clumping of blood platelets. These drugs do not require constant laboratory monitoring as do anticoagulants.

Medication to help lower risk factors treating hyperlipidemia
The importance of treating risk factors such as obesity with dietary measures is no longer disputed. It is recommended that not only the normal weight, but the ideal weight be attained in order to control hyperlipoproteinemia (elevated fat levels in the blood), hyperuricemia (elevated uric acid levels), diabetes and hypertension. If the elevated cholesterol levels (above 260mg%) cannot be reduced by dieting, certain drugs depending on the type of hyperlipoproteinemia such as clofibrate or cholestyramine may be prescribed.

Abnormal fat levels in the blood

Treating hyperuricemia
Elevated uric acid levels in the blood are treated with drugs which reduce these levels even if these have not resulted in gout, the formation of kidney stones or any other symptoms. In men the normal uric acid level is 7mg%, and in women it is 6mg%.

Elevated uric acid levels

Treating hypertension
Drug therapy for hypertension is an important, but also complex, issue.
The patient should be made aware of the fact that effective

Medication for hypertensives

treatment of hypertension causes temporary symptoms of hypotension (low blood pressure), because the central nervous system cannot immediately adjust to a sudden lowering of blood pressure. The drug treatment makes the hypertensive a hypotensive patient with symptoms of fatigue and dizziness. However, this phase lasts only a few weeks until the body becomes accustomed to the normotensive level. It is important to inform the patient of the effects of this phase because unfortunately many patients stop taking the medication and thus create a potentially dangerous situation for themselves. An important observation is worth repeating here: "Hypertension causes no symptoms but does cause death whereas hypotension causes symptoms but not death." The blood pressure should not

Proper dosage is important

be lowered abruptly to the normal value of 120/80mmHg. For more details you should consult your physician (see also p. 24).

Since effective drugs are available to treat hypertension, other measures are often neglected. These measures are, however, important because a salt-free diet which is also low in calories and diuretics play a significant role.

Medication to encourage weight loss

Dangerous consequences

The patient ought to be warned that some of the drugs to curb the appetite cause serious side-effects (for example, increased pressure in the pulmonary circulation) and have therefore been removed from the market.

We would like to end this section in the way we began it by stressing compliance which determines the success of any long-term drug therapy. The continued research on pharmaceuticals, combined with the patient's understanding and motivation is of equal importance.

Eating What the Heart Desires

When we saw one of our colleagues again after long period of time, we were surprised to see how well-rested and slim he looked, especially when he told us that he had sustained a heart attack. He conceded that after the heart attack he had finally undertaken all the measures he should have taken to prevent it and quit smoking, lost thirty-five pounds, took more vacations and began to hike again. As a result, he now felt better than he had prior to the heart attack.

Lose weight immediately

Dr. R. M. had begun to lose weight immediately after the heart attack by restricting himself to a one thousand calorie diet. In our experience, however, we have found that heart attack patients often gain weight because they tend to eat more than they should during their confinement to bed.

Overweight often triggers other risk factors such as abnormal fat levels in the blood, hypertension, diabetes and elevated uric acid levels (hyperuricemia). Overweight also leads to lack of physical activity because it is more difficult to exercise with excess weight. After a heart attack every pound which is lost reduces the patient's risks and improves his condition, plus allowing him to recover more quickly by decreasing the work-load of the myocardium. The patient must accept the fact that rehabilitation begins with normalizing the weight and he should have the ideal weight as his goal. (See the Weight Chart on p. 95. Ideal weight is the lower figure in your weight category. For example, the ideal weight for a medium framed man of 6 feet is 154 pounds.)

Making it easier for the heart to work

Determining your ideal weight

In the Western industrialized countries, one out of three persons is overweight. Perhaps you are also one of the adults who consumes more than 3,000 calories per day and thus takes in 600 to 800 more calories than the body requires. Perhaps you have not admitted to yourself that you are overweight and react defensively, asking "Where is the pot-belly?" and exclaiming, "Then I would be only skin and bones!" upon seeing how much you should weigh. If overweight patients are asked what they think their normal weight should be, they usually underestimate it considerably. About 10% of the patients who are 20% overweight consider themselves to be normal weight and another 10% of the patients believe that they have particularly heavy bones which in themselves weigh 88 pounds. Actually, a skeleton weighs between 17 and 22 pounds. If you have decided after your heart attack to lose weight, perhaps with the cooperation of your spouse, you should understand why the following excuses which are frequently heard, are false.

"Fat protects the nerves."

False excuses
The fact that there are both overweight and normal weight

94

Weight Chart

	Small Frame	Medium Frame	Large Frame
Weight in pounds in indoor clothing, with shoes.			
Men (over age 25)			
5'2"	112-120	118-129	126-141
5'4"	118-126	124-136	132-148
5'6"	124-133	130-143	138-156
5'8"	132-141	138-152	147-166
5'10"	140-150	146-160	155-174
6'0"	148-158	154-170	164-184
6'2"	156-167	162-180	173-194
6'4"	164-175	172-190	182-204
Women (Over age 25)			
4'10"	92-98	96-107	104-119
5'0"	96-104	101-113	109-125
5'2"	102-110	107-119	115-131
5'4"	108-116	113-126	121-138
5'6"	114-123	120-135	129-146
5'8"	122-131	128-143	137-154
5'10"	130-140	136-151	145-163

Relaxing through eating?

persons who are either nervous or calm shows that slimness is not necessarily correlated with being nervous. Eating can have a calming, relaxing effect, but when it leads to overweight it is not a suitable way of reducing tension. Even if you are a little more restless on a diet than you usually are, this discomfort is only temporary and well worth the end result. Perhaps you should experiment with ways other than eating to relax. If you ask former obese patients about the effects of weight loss, they will probably tell you that they are now more active, agile, productive, and more enterprising than previously.

Reserve fat is an extra load

"One has to have spare fat!"
This belief appeared to be valid up to the early part of our

95

century when regional wars, meager harvests and infectious diseases such as tuberculosis were still great risk factors. However, tuberculosis can be treated effectively and extra layers of fat offer no protection from atomic weapons or emaciating diseases such as cancer. Overweight is simply an additional risk factor for heart attacks and other diseases common in civilized countries.

"My overweight is hereditary and besides, my hormones do not function properly."
The cause of overweight is almost always overeating, but is rarely due to hereditary factors or hormones as is frequently claimed. Some persons, of course, do utilize what they eat better than others, but in the vast majority of cases, overweight is the result of excessive caloric intake. The phrase *eating too much* is relative, but it is nonetheless clear that the excess fat deposited on the belly or hips was taken in through the mouth. If you eat more than you can expend in working calories, you gain weight, and conversely, you lose weight if you eat less than your body needs.

Obese persons overeat

"My overweight is due to lack of exercise."
Physical activity has doubtless many advantages for your health and also helps heart attack patients overcome depressions. However, since the body uses calories sparingly, you must walk six miles to use up the calories contained in a hot fudge sundae.

A bottle of beer equals an eight mile hike

Caloric Expenditure (30 Minutes)	
Walking 1¼ mi/hr	51 calories
Bicycling 6¼ mi/hr	84 calories
Walking 3mi/hr	94 calories
Gymnastics	150 calories
Playing golf	155 calories
Dancing the fox trot	156 calories
Playing table tennis	165 calories
Paddling 410ft.	204 calories
Dancing the rhumba	210 calories
Cross country skiing, 2½ mi/hr	240 calories
Snow shoveling	250 calories
Swimming breast stroke 164ft/min	340 calories

"I have tried to lose weight several times unsuccessfully."

*Did you
really try?*

There is only one explanation for this excuse, that you have not realized (or may not want to realize) that your method for losing weight was wrong.

"It is dangerous to lose weight after a heart attack."
On the contrary, common sense tells us that the heart of an obese person is in all respects at a greater disadvantage than the heart of a normal weight person.

● Since the additional adipose fat tissue must also be supplied with oxygen, the heart is forced to pump more blood.

● When an overweight person exercises, his excessive fat is as much a burden as an extra back-pack. His heart has to work like a Volkswagen engine in a Mac truck.

● The heart is also at a disadvantage because movement of the diaphragm in the act of breathing is impaired and pressure in the pulmonary arteries rises.

● Fat deposits in the sac surrounding the heart muscle impede the contractions of the myocardium.

Are you still not convinced that excess fat adds a burden to the heart?

Unfortunately, excess weight does not disappear by itself after a heart attack as is often assumed. A study by Drs. Gillman and Colberg showed that patients who were twenty pounds overweight had not attained their normal weight in the five-year observation period after the heart attack and that one-third of the patients actually gained more weight.

*How to lose
weight*

How can excess weight be lost? The answer sounds very simple: you should eat a little less than your body actually needs every day. Your diet should consist of fewer calories, but should not be extreme in any respect and should take all your risk factors into consideration. Dr. H. Anemueller calls this a "heart protective diet", while some call it a "prudent diet" and still others call it an "ideal diet". The ideal diet for a heart attack patient is ideal also for other persons, whether they are young or old, healthy or sick. The entire family should participate in this diet.

We have decided to include only the theoretical basis of the ideal diet and to refer you to a special book, a classic, with great recipes: Dr. Ancel Keys, *Eat Well—Stay Well."* (Doubleday, New York, 1963).

You should avoid foods which are rich in calories, but are not nutritious and choose instead those foods which contain few calories. Such foods will not only satisfy your hunger, but also contain essential minerals and vitamins. You should begin by writing down everything you eat and drink over a period of three days. Then you should add up the number of calories and calculate your average caloric intake. Most persons with average physical activity can successfully lose weight if they reduce their caloric intake to 1,200 per day and weigh themselves daily. Your body will compensate for a diet containing few calories by using up adipose fat tissue. As a rule of thumb, 2.2 pounds contain 6,000 calories. In summary, if you observe the following rules, you will certainly lose weight:

First calculate your calorie intake

Basic rules for losing weight

- Do not consume more than 1,200 calories until your weight becomes normalized.
- Consume as few fats as possible. Your dietary cookbooks which are available from your local American Heart Association will indicate those foods which are high in fats and will warn you about foods which contain hidden fats.
- Restrict your carbohydrate intake. Carbohydrates are transformed into fats in the body, and are found in bread, noodles, flour, rice, potatoes, and all foods containing sugar, as well as in soft drinks and alcohol. You should note that a glass of wine or beer contains 90 to 120 calories.
- Since salt retains body fluid, you should attempt to substitute herbs and spices for salt as often as possible (see page 123).
- Consume an adequate amount of protein, preferably in a form which contains few calories.
- Should you be disappointed with your weight loss because you overate on a single day, then fast for a day. For best results, fast one day per week, drinking only low caloric fluids during that day.
- Weigh yourself daily before breakfast, without clothing, and keep a record of your weight.

In most hospitals, you may request a special diet of 800 to 1,000 calories per day. Ask your physician about this in order to make a good start on your weight loss either in the hospital or at the rehabilitation clinic.

A healthier diet.

Heart attacks are caused in part not only by excessive caloric intake, but also by the poor quality of the diet. Both of these factors play an important role in obesity because the more a person consumes of an unhealthy diet, the more weight he will gain. The less a person eats, the less is the chance that he is eating the wrong food. A healthy diet also plays an important role in reducing and eliminating the various risk factors, such as abnormal fat levels in the blood, diabetes, hypertension, and hyperuricemia.

Fats. The majority of cases involving abnormal fat levels in the blood can be corrected with appropriate changes in the diet. An effective and lasting reduction of cholesterol levels probably greatly lowers the risk of heart attack. Which fats in our diet are harmful? How is it possible that one in five adults and 10% of

Fatty Acid Content of Different Fats (in percent)

Fats	Saturated Fatty Acids	Monounsaturated Fatty Acids	Polyunsaturated Fatty Acids
Coconut Fat	92	6	2
Palm Oil	46	44	10
Cotton Seed Oil	25	25	50
Olive Oil	19	73	8
Peanut Oil	19	50	31
Safflower Oil	10	15	75
Sunflower Seed Oil	8	27	65
Corn Oil	8	27	65
Soya Bean Oil	14	24	62
Butter	60	37	3
Lard	43	49	8
Margarine: Excellent Quality	25	25	50
Poor Quality	50	20	30

school children already have elevated lipid levels?

We not only eat too much fat, but we also consume the wrong fats. Fats consist of fatty acids, which are either:
- Poly-unsaturated, mono-unsaturated, or
- Saturated fatty acids.

The desirable poly-unsaturated fatty acids are mostly found in vegetable fats and oils, while saturated fatty acids are contained mainly in animal fats (see table). However, there are exceptions: as the table indicates, at least two vegetable oils (coconut oil and palm oil) have an extremely high percentage of saturated fatty

acids and are, therefore, undesirable. Margarines of poor quality used to contain a considerable amount of coconut oil, but the most recently developed margarines are of improved quality since primarily poly-unsaturated fatty acids are utilized in their production. On the other hand, fish oil is composed of more poly-unsaturated and mono-unsaturated fat than of saturated fat. This is one reason why it would be desirable to increase the fish consumption in the American diet to two or three dinners per week. It is known that any excess in fat intake is deposited as body fat. Theoretically, not more than 60 to 70 grams (or 2 to 2½ ounces) of fat should be consumed per day. You should take into consideration not only the visible fats (salad oil, and fats in cooking, spreading, frying and baking), but also invisible fats (found in convenience foods from vending machines, TV dinners, packaged meats, sausages, milk products and all processed foods). Heart attack patients should consume as little fat as possible and take advantage of fat-free cooking methods such as broiling and cooking on a grill or in an aluminum foil or roasting bag. Always cook, bake or fry with margarine and vegetable oils (sunflower, corn, soya bean, or safflower oil).

How much cholesterol is permissible in your diet? As you know, cholesterol is found in hormones and can be produced by the body without actual intake of cholesterol. Since the body produces 1,000 to 4,000 milligrams per day, you should restrict the dietary cholesterol intake as much as possible. If you wish to keep your cholesterol level low, you should first of all restrict your total calorie and fat intake, and then pay particular attention to the dietary cholesterol intake by reducing it from the usual 600 milligrams to 300. You ought to take into account that one egg yolk alone contains almost 300 milligrams of cholesterol. Avoid foods rich in cholesterol such as eggs, butter, lard, shrimp, as well as inner organ meats such as kidney, liver, and brain.

If you reduce or eliminate your intake of inner organ meats, fat, sauces, meat broths and extracts, salt meat, sausage and shrimp, you will also lower your uric acid level and thus reduce the risk factor of hyperuricemia. If this is one of your problems, you should try to reach and then maintain your normal weight. You should also be aware of the fact that alcohol plays a significant role in hyperuricemia. The following foods are suitable for a low purine-free diet, which helps to reduce hyperuricemia: milk and milk products, margarine, oil, all kinds of fruits and fruit juices, bread, starches, potatoes, rice, green salad, tomatoes, radishes, cucumbers, all cabbages, beets, pumpkin, celery, carrots, and onions (however, vegetables such as asparagus, spinach, and dried beans and peas are relatively rich in purine).

Purine-free foods

Carbohydrates. We obtain most of our calories from this group of foods which includes fruits, vegetables, rice, corn, and flour products such as bread, cake, and noodles. Carbohydrates resemble fats in that they are also good energy-providers. Since most people who tend to gain weight like the taste of various carbohydrates, they are overweight as a result of excessive carbohydrate intake. Carbohydrates should be consumed in moderation because any excess intake is converted into body fat. Like alcohol, carbohydrates elevate the triglyceride levels. If an elevated triglyceride level is one of your risk factors, you should restrict your intake of carbohydrates, and in particular, of sugar and alcohol. Moreover, carbohydrates elevate the blood sugar level, a fact of particular importance to diabetics. Fortunately, however, not all carbohydrates have the same effect. The table on page 102 shows that some carbohydrates such as sugar and soft drinks shoot into the blood and other such as bread, starches and potatoes stream into the blood while carbohydrates made from milk products and vegetables seep slowly into the blood. This difference of absorption rate within the carbohydrate group indicates the difference in the speed with which blood sugar is elevated. In their book, *Risk Factors of Ischemic Heart Disease,* Drs. S. Heyden and G. Wolff describe what happens when an overweight person finishes his breakfast consisting of two pieces of toast, jam and coffee with sugar: in the fasting state his blood sugar of 97mg% is still within the normal limit. But within half an hour after this breakfast rich in carbohydrates, the blood sugar

Watch carbohydrate intake

When the blood sugar decreases sharply

101

level shoots up to 185mg%. This blood sugar elevation does not constitute diabetes, but it is higher than the upper normal limit, usually set at 150mg%, thirty minutes after the carbohydrate-rich meal. This condition is called hyperglycemia. Insulin should have prevented the rise of the blood sugar to such a high level but it was not available right when it was needed. It is typical for overweight patients to show a sort of resistance to insulin, at least temporarily. The blood sugar, however, does not remain elevated. Insulin appears in a belated response to decrease the hyperglycemic blood level. The pancreas now pours insulin into the blood, causing the blood sugar to plunge down to 65mg% in the following two hours. When the blood sugar falls sharply, the patient experiences various complaints such as headaches which do not respond to medication, fatigue, restlessness, perspiration, irritation, and most importantly, he is very hungry. Most overweight persons feel that something is wrong and have a strong desire to eat more carbohydrates in the belief that this will relieve their discomfort. Thus, an overweight person who consumes a meal rich in carbohydrates is satisfied for three or four hours, at which time he becomes very hungry again. Since he will then consume more food, it is not surprising that he will gain more weight.

How the body absorbs carbohydrates

1. Sugar, soft drinks — shoot into the blood

2. Starches, bread, potatoes — stream into the blood

3. Fruits — flow into the blood

4. Carbohydrates made from milk — drip into the blood

5. Vegetables — seep into the blood

Carbohydrates which quickly shoot into the blood also play an important role in the diet of a diabetic. The diabetic should carefully calculate his carbohydrate intake and make certain that it does not exceed his body's actual need. The sugar metabolism may be stabilized in all persons, not only in diabetics, by choosing a diet rich in whole grain and whole wheat products rather than in products made from refined sugar and bleached flour. We cannot describe the diet of a diabetic in detail, but we would like to point out that many overweight persons who develop diabetes in old age, may become non-diabetics again by simply losing thirty to forty pounds.

Protein. The body uses protein to rebuild body tissue. Red blood cells have a life span of 120 days—then they die. In order to build new red blood cells, protein is needed since it is the most important building block of each cell. If not enough protein is provided in the food intake, anemia is one of the consequences. Significant lack of protein is a common problem only in the third world, but not in the U.S. or in Central European countries. Protein is found in milk and milk products, eggs, meat and fish, as well as in nuts, peas and dried beans, mushrooms, and grain products. The intake of protein should not exceed the body's demand of protein which is one gram per 2¼ pounds of body weight daily. An excessive intake of protein is useless and too rich in purine and accompanying fats. You should be careful to choose those foods which are rich in protein, but low in fats.

Salt: A diet rich in salt poses an additional danger for the heart and circulation because it can lead to hypertension and fluid retention. You should consume as little salt as possible. However, a low salt diet does not necessarily taste bad because various herbs may be used to spice a meal. A good cookbook will show how herbs and spices such as the following may be used: lemon, parsley, scallions, chive, garlic, horse radish, capers, juniper berries, unsalted yeast extract, low-sodium mustard, and low-sodium catsup, as well as anis, basil, curry, dill, fennel, caraway seed, bay leaves, marjoram, nutmeg, clove, pepper, sage, rosemary, thyme, paprika, onion and garlic powder. A large variety of meals can be cooked with the herbs and spices mentioned. The appendix on p. 123 should be of great help.

Are alcohol, coffee, or tea permissible?

Is alcohol as harmful as smoking? Or does alcohol dilate the vessels, so that the heart is not burdened? If your liver is healthy and you are moderate in your alcohol consumption, alcohol will not cause any harm to your body. Many persons do not know how much they may drink safely, and the amount is lower than many believe. Alcohol consumption may not only make it difficult to lose weight, but will also cause liver damage if more than 2½ ounces are consumed daily. This amount is found in only five beers (each with a 4½% alcohol content).

Alcohol is not a thirst quencher

Many heart attack patients tolerate coffee and do not experience irregular cardiac rhythm or elevated blood pressure when they drink it. Others become restless, feel that their heart rate is irregular, and think that coffee elevates the blood pressure, especially when they take their own blood pressure at home. The question about coffee can only be answered individually but not in a general fashion. We urge each patient to experiment in order to discover how many cups of coffee he can tolerate without experiencing side-effects. Neither coffee nor tea is a risk factor for heart attack. Studies which claim to prove that coffee and tea are harmful have not been controlled for cigarette smoking and are therefore unreliable.

From Smoker to Ex-Smoker.

Of those who develop a heart attack, almost 90% are smokers. Since smoking is clearly a risk factor for heart attack, 60% of the patients stop smoking altogether, while 30% stop smoking only for a short period of time. We know from our experiences that those who start smoking again are depressed about it and we also realize how difficult a second attempt to stop smoking can be.

Stopping for good

Is it really imperative that the coronary patient quit smoking? The answer is "yes" without any reservation. All excuses such as smoking "only one cigarette in the evening," smoking cigarettes low in nicotine, or smoking through a special filter, are unjustifiable. Reducing the number to three or five cigarettes per day is self-deception. The price of smoking is too high because it will certainly lead to re-infarction.

There are no "health" filters

In healthy persons we do not condemn an occasional cigarette, but in the case of patients with myocardial infarction, we must

104

insist that smoking poses a serious threat. In our experience, continued cigarette smoking is a significant factor in fatal re-infarction.

You should take advantage of the no-smoking rule in the intensive care unit and the hospital in order to become accustomed to never touching another cigarette. If you did not take this opportunity seriously, there is another chance in the rehabilitation center. In such surroundings where all patients are urged to quit smoking and where the patient is not tempted to smoke as he may be at his work site or at home, it is relatively easy even for chain-smokers to quit. The transitional stage is easier for the patient if he participates in the anti-smoking groups, physical therapy, diet, and special program of exercise

administered by experienced and qualified therapists. Most of the rehabilitation centers for heart attack patients offer anti-smoking groups which give the patient a good second chance to quit.

If you are in the intensive care unit or hospital while reading this book, there is only one thing you can do: never smoke another cigarette! Any advice to the contrary is against your best interest. The following suggestions should make it easier for you to stop smoking.

Aids to help you quit smoking

Sports. Physical activity can have the same effect as smoking a cigarette by stimulating a person who is tired and exhausted, and relaxing a person who is nervous. Sports may play a significant role in helping a person to quit smoking, particularly in the beginning.

Sleep. To insure your success in stopping smoking, you should
always get sufficient sleep, taking a nap in the afternoon if necessary, because when you are tired, you are more likely to reach for a cigarette. To avoid falling back into your old habit pattern, you should try not to tire yourself out. If you have trouble sleeping in the transition period, you should take a sleeping pill.

Variety. Boredom leads to smoking in the same way fatigue and stress do. You should diversify your leisure time activities by seeing a movie, exhibition, or play, by attending a lecture, or going to a concert. Try to find a book or hobby which interests you.

Relaxation. Yoga and related methods can greatly help a person to quit smoking, but are not usually emphasized as strongly as they should. Yoga can make persons more aware of certain body processes, behavior patterns and environmental factors. The person then gains the ability to influence his surroundings and himself in such a way as to make it easier to finally quit his smoking habit.

You should not learn yoga on your own because you may then develop certain undesirable habits which are difficult to correct. We suggest instead that you join a group or take a course offered by your clinic, university or in your city.

Change of diet. All who have tried to quit smoking, but then gained 10 pounds, know that smoking and eating are closely related. A variety of reasons have been suggested to explain why non-smokers generally eat and therefore weigh more than smokers, and also why ex-smokers gain weight so easily. It is clear that cigarettes have a direct influence on the digestive system and also that a smoker gets oral satisfaction from a cigarette while a non-smoker satisfies himself with food.

Oral satisfaction through eating?

Since overweight is one of the risk factors, you should be careful not to gain weight after your heart attack by checking it regularly.

Develop a preference for fruits and salads

Seventh-Day Adventists offer a five-day plan to stop smoking and have discovered that smokers in general do not eat much salad or many fruits. It seems, however, that a diet rich in raw vegetables and fruits, but low in meat and fish makes it easier to stop smoking. I can offer no explanation for why this plan works, but can only urge you to try it. This plan has the additional advantage of helping patients overcome constipation if they have that tendency. Laxatives may be more convenient, but an addiction to laxatives can cause irreversible damage. When laxatives are taken simultaneously with drugs to lower the blood pressure (diurectics), they may cause a significant potassium deficiency. It would be better to change the dietary habits as described in the section "Eating What Your Heart Desires" (page 93).

Drink more than usual

The five-day plan also advocates that patients who are trying to stop smoking drink more than they usually would. They do not mean, of course, that the patient should drink more alcohol. Since many smokers are also heavy coffee drinkers, it is also suggested that the patients who are trying to stop smoking drink less coffee or temporarily switch to tea, in order to break their old habit pattern.

106

Why should the patients drink more? A theory suggests that people should drink more to replace oral satisfaction of a cigarette.

Begin your day by drinking two glasses of fruit juice, warm milk, water, or tea before breakfast. Between meals, you could drink water, lemonade, juice, or milk, but you should always take care to restrict your caloric intake from these drinks.

Oral satisfaction

Smoking clearly has something to do with oral satisfaction. In the transition period, many patients try to replace the cigarette in their mouth with chewing gum or candy. You should not, however, indiscriminately substitute chocolate, sweets, sandwiches or salted nuts for the cigarette because you will gain weight immediately.

Instead, those who need oral satisfaction may chew on the end of a cigarette holder or the tip of a menthol cigarette. You should always have some chewing gum with you, or dietary bonbons, licorice, peppermints, sour drops and anything that leaves a pleasant taste in your mouth. You also could suck on dried fruits with pits for many hours.

Some anti-smoking clinics offer radishes, cucumber, carrots, celery, and whole wheat crackers, as well as mixed pickles and home-made popcorn.

But is there no medication to help you quit smoking? We certainly wish that such medication would be available to our patients, but none has yet been developed, even though certain magazines and newspapers proclaim that there are such drugs.

Do not take drugs to help you stop smoking

Although we discuss anti-smoking drugs in one chapter of our book on smoking, and recommend some of them to healthy persons, we do not advise our heart patients to take them since they may cause undesirable side effects. The patient with myocardial infarction should not take any risk with such drugs, especially since he should be more motivated to quit smoking, having learned a lesson from the heart attack.

Withdrawal symptoms and how to overcome them

Withdrawal symptoms

Our experience has shown that patients most easily stop smoking and experience the least number of withdrawal symptoms if they

107

quit right after having sustained a heart attack. However, if withdrawal symptoms do occur, they may be classified and treated as one of the following three types:

● Problems resulting from the lack of oral gratification which may cause, for example, increased appetite and weight gain.

● Problems related to the lack of physical-emotional stimulation resulting, for example, in fatigue, listlessness, difficulty in concentrating or impaired circulation.

● Examples of the inability to calm down include problems such as higher pulse rate, irritability, restlessness, nervousness and insomnia.

Stimulate body and mind

In order to alleviate these discomforts, you should find something to substitute for the function of the cigarette that you are missing. Thus if your problems are related to the lack of stimulation you should find some kind of sports or game which is as stimulating to you as the cigarette. If, however, you are nervous, restless, irritable and suffer from insomnia, then your problems are related to the tranquilizing effect which a cigarette may have. In this case, you should experiment with a meaningful program of exercise and yoga. Sometimes sedatives or tranquilizers are necessary during the transitional period. You should discuss your complaints with your physician and ask him to write a prescription for you (possibly Valium or Librium).

Balanced Exercise That Is Fun

The title of this important section stresses our concern that exercise should be balanced. In this section we shall discuss exercise in general and later we shall take into consideration the kind of training and sports in which you may participate.

Why exercise is so important

Why is exercise important for the coronary heart patient following the heart attack? Let us begin with the negative aspects of the lack of exercise. Even in a healthy person, a two-week-long period of confinement to bed can lead to 25% loss of muscle tone and to an equal reduction in the ability of the body to utilize oxygen. After prolonged bed rest, even a healthy person must breathe more frequently and requires a higher pulse rate to perform even minor physical activities.

On the other hand, physical therapy administered in the

hospital as part of early mobilization improves the circulation to the muscles, the coordination of the central nervous system and the skeletal muscles, and also promotes the functional adaptation of various organs.

The work load of the heart is effectively reduced when the interplay of muscle tone is improved because then less blood oxygen must be pumped to the muscles. The heart rate decreases and the respiratory rate becomes less rapid.

Better care for the heart

Such a heart has its function "economized", relieved of excess work load as a result of physical therapy, but only if the exercise is balanced. The physician determines how much exercise may be tolerated on the basis of recovery rate and diagnostic tests such as ergometry. If you participate in a coronary exercise group, the physician can prescribe the suitable amount of exercise by checking your pulse, the development of complaints, and irregularities of cardiac rhythm in the course of physical therapy.

If you should walk, hike, and then perhaps jog on your own, you should be careful not to allow your pulse to exceed 110 beats per minute during the first few weeks. Later your maximum pulse should be adjusted to your age. A convenient rule of thumb is that your pulse rate should equal 180 minus your age (for example, the pulse of a person 60 years of age should not exceed 120 beats per minute). The success of balanced exercise can be measured already after a few weeks in a bicycle ergometer test. The pulse will have decreased and the blood pressure risen when it is compared to previous tests.

Exercise therapy and sports for the coronary patient
The most appropriate exercises are those which involve the greatest number of muscles for at least three minutes, and thus influence peripheral circulation. The more economical and the better the peripheral circulation, the less demand there is for oxygen and the less work the heart must perform. We must insist on this point because it is often incorrectly assumed that physical therapy increases the work load of the heart. We highly recommend endurance exercises such as prolonged walking, strolling, jogging (while jogging you should be able to continue a conversation with your fellow jogger), running, bicycle riding, cross country skiing, and swimming.

Improved circulation

109

Which exercises should be avoided?

All exercises which involve forced breathing such as lifting and hoisting, push-ups, sprinting, and diving should be avoided.

Our experience has shown that swimming should be allowed in water of 80 degrees Fahrenheit only when the patient is capable of attaining 75 watts for six minutes on a bicycle ergometer test without showing subjective or objective signs of coronary insufficiency or irregular cardiac rhythm. To avoid forced breathing, only those patients who swim well and like to swim should be allowed to do so.

It must be
fun

Moreover, exercise should be fun, because the psychological effects are at least as important as the physical ones for the coronary patients. Patients gain self-confidence and "joie de vivre" when they are able to increase their physical activity and overcome previous limitations. At the same time, fears that exist, but are not expressed, diminish in strength. In this respect exercise is an important part of psychotherapy.

Avoid
competitive
sports

Patients who tend to be over-achievers must be made aware of the playful nature of exercise, because they should not be forcing themselves, or gritting the teeth to get the exercising done. We must also warn patients about competitive sports which could cause over-exertion. Thus we can recommend tennis only to those who play for fun, but not to those who insist on winning.

In concluding this section, we would like to stress that any kind of exercise performed regularly contributes to reduction of risk factors. Thus, as the blood pressure is lowered and weight loss is made easier, the fat levels are also normalized. Moreover, the danger of hyperuricemia and the formation of blood clots is reduced, and the abnormal carbohydrate metabolism of diabetics can be much improved.

Adjusting to Stress

If we accept the hypothesis that so-called psychosocial stress in occupation and personal relationships is a contributing factor to coronary heart disease, then we must agree that there are two ways of overcoming such stress:

● reducing or eliminating the stressors or
● reducing the reaction to stressors, in other words, learning to adapt.

Change or
learn to
adjust

When it is not possible to change the situations which cause stress, the reaction to the stressors should be changed. We shall briefly mention a few ways, but must leave to the individual the responsibility of discovering the most suitable method for himself. Such methods range from medication (like beta blockers) to yoga for relaxation, from behavior therapy (anti-smoking clinics) to group therapy (marriage counseling), and toward developing a new philosophy of life and changing one's attitude about the world and life situations in general.

Every patient should reappraise his system of values while in the hospital or while in early rehabilitation. We highly recommend that younger and more ambitious patients evaluate their life-styles

Establishing a
new life-style

in order to determine whether their hopes and wishes have been fulfilled. In our discussion groups we often asked former coronary patients what was the most important thing they learned in the clinic. One related that he learned to enjoy exercise, another that he quit smoking. A construction worker once told us that he finally learned not to let people or things bother him any more.

We are not exaggerating when we note that many coronary patients lead a happier and more fulfilled life after the heart attack, because they finally learn to enjoy life and to face it with greater appreciation and gratitude. The analogy with the wine glass is appropriate here, because certainly the optimist who says the glass is half-full will be happier than the pessimist who says that it is half-empty.

10. Assistance for a Second Life

Partnership and Sexuality

A problem that affects patient and spouse

If we are concerned not only in saving the life of heart attack patients, but also in helping them recover physically and emotionally, then we must also take sexuality into consideration. In our discussion groups, we found that few physicians mention sex and that patients rarely receive the detailed information they hope to obtain. In our group, two-thirds of the patients had not received information about sex after the heart attack and one-third obtained either vague incorrect information or prohibitions against such activity.

Another observation which coincides with this one is that the sexual habits of many patients who have recovered from a heart attack differ considerably from their habits prior to the attack. They live as though they were twenty years older in their sexual habits, although they no longer experience complaints, perform well in a bicycle ergometer test, and have returned to their former jobs and social life.

Swiss and American studies show that one year after the heart attack, two-thirds of the patients had greatly decreased their sexual activity and that the remaining one-third of the patients had no further sexual contact.

Our male patients often relate a considerable decrease in their libido and potency, and thus experience fewer intimate contacts.

Discussion groups with wives of heart attack patients reveal that older women react either with resignation because the situation seems beyond their control, or with a sense of relief because they are no longer required to fulfill an unpleasant duty. However, younger wives of a generation in which sexual desires are expressed more openly often declare that they do not intend to give up sex.

112

Problems with libido and potency

Where the problems may lie

What are the causes of the problems with libido and potency experienced by younger and middle-aged men who have recovered completely from their heart attacks? Three major causes which can be treated by the general practitioner or a specialist, must be discussed.

1. Problems with potency may result from impaired peripheral circulation. Those risk factors which lead to a heart attack also cause changes in the blood circulation of other organs. For

Vessel changes

example, heavy smoking results in changes in the arteries of the pelvic area and legs. Such impaired circulation could be responsible for the insufficient oxygen supply of the sexual organs which would lead in turn to impotence. Impaired circulation may be the cause of your problems if you answer the following questions in the affirmative.

● Do you feel that your libido has not changed but that you simply have problems with erection?

● Have you noticed a sense of fatigue and heaviness in your legs when you walk, which sometimes leads to cramps in your calf muscles?

● Does such pain appear when you climb stairs quickly? Does the pain disappear if you stand still for a few minutes?

In this case you should request that your physician make the necessary arrangements to evaluate your peripheral circulation. He may send you to an angiologist, a specialist in vascular diseases. With an anteriography, using a contrast material injected into the blood vessels, minute details of the vessels can be examined. The body can compensate for unilateral occlusions in blood vessels, but bilateral occlusions lead to problems with penile erection. If these occlusions are to be removed, your physician will put you in contact with a vascular surgeon who can inform you about the risks, means, and types of blood vessel surgery. The chances for a successful surgery are about 70%.

2. Impotence may result from the medication which heart attack patients must take. Such drugs include almost all those which lower blood pressure, some which influence the fat metabolism,

Side-effects of drugs may be the cause

many tranquilizers, and several anti-depressants. It is difficult to give precise information about all the drugs, because there exist anti-depressants which may, for example, enhance potency.

113

Besides, the drugs are prescribed for a specific reason, and some must be taken for life, as for example, those which lower blood pressure. We do not want the patient to suddenly stop taking his medication because he read in this book that it could cause impotence. Therefore, we must emphasize that medication can sometimes be one of the cause of impotence, but it does not in general lead to this result.

How should one proceed if all the causes of impotence can be eliminated, except for the drug against hypertension? In this case we would try different medications. However, since it is rather unlikely that we would be able to determine the exact drug and combination of factors which cause impotence, it would probably be easier to treat the hypertension in a different way. For example, the patient could check his own blood pressure regularly, lose more weight, intensify his exercise, or take dietary measures such as restricting his salt intake.

Fortunately, there are not only drugs which impair potency, but also those which enhance it. In many cases the undesirable side-effects of one drug can be balanced against the desirable side-effects of others. One of the most important drugs for heart attack patients, the nitrates and anticoagulants, can increase potency through improved erection and orgasm as the chest pains disappear. This is another reason for prescribing nitrates generously and taking them regularly.

Basic emotional problems may be the cause

3. The major cause of impotence after a heart attack is an emotional one rather than a physical one. Is it not surprising and perhaps symptomatic of our scientific medicine that the emotional processes leading to a heart attack and its emotional effects are discussed so rarely?

Secret fears
Lack of time is not the only reason for the fact that sex is so rarely discussed between the patient and the physician. Rather, this silence is caused by the fact that most of the patients and physicians have lived in a generation which makes sexual questions taboo. Thus, secret fears of the heart attack patient are not expressed, so they cannot be treated and may have a harmful effect on his sex life in the future. In private and confidential discussions with our patients, we have been able to determine and

114

allay many of these apprehensions.

What do patients fear? They are primarily anxious that the emotional and physical exertion of intercourse could harm their hearts. Could the stress, the increased pulse and respiratory rate not cause a new heart attack? The spouse, of course, shares this secret fear with the patient, but neither partner may like to discuss it. The more severe the heart attack was, the more difficult it is for the patient and spouse to talk about this anxiety. Often, not only the patient and spouse, but also the physician is ill at ease. He may also tend to overestimate the physical and emotional exertion of intercourse. Unfortunately, little information is available to the patient and the physician about this important topic.

The American cardiologists Hellerstein and Friedman observed the long-term EKG's of forty-eight heart attack and forty-three coronary heart disease patients over 24- to 28-hour periods. The patients performed their daily activities but did not know that the physicians were primarily interested in their sexual activity. It was found that the average pulse reading during an orgasm was 117 beats per minute. The highest rate was 144 and the lowest 90 beats per minute. Two minutes before and after the orgasm, the heart rate was 97 beats per minute.

In order to interpret these numbers they must be compared to the heart rates and electrocardiographic changes of other activities and the bicycle ergometric test. The findings of a 44-year-old business man were typical for most patients: the increase of the heart rate was higher when he worked, drove his car, participated in a heated discussion and played ball with his son than it was during intercourse. Thus the increase in heart rate, respiration, and blood pressure during coitus corresponds to the increase experienced when producing 75 watts in the bicycle ergometer test. Therefore, a patient may resume his sexual activities without harm if he is able to generate 75 watts in the ergometer, quickly climb a flight of stairs or walk around a block quickly without major complaints.

The patient should also resume his sexual activity because studies on sex in old age have revealed that nothing is as detrimental to intercourse in the second half of life as the breaking of habits. If weeks, months, or even years pass since the last intercourse, then it is much harder to resume such activity.

We therefore recommend that patients renew their sexual

contacts as soon as they leave the hospital and can return to their daily activities. But what happens if complaints develop? Such complaints must be carefully examined because some, such as palpitations, occur even in healthy persons during intercourse and should not cause concern. If the patient develops true anginal pain as described on page 34 and which is also caused by any other physical activity, then he should know which measures he must take after having read this book. On page 88, we recommended that nitrates should be taken to prevent complaints which develop during physical exertion. We make the same suggestion for anginal pain which arises when you are in bed. You should keep nitrates close at hand and take them as a preventive measure before engaging in sexual activity.

Palpitations are no cause for concern

Some patients are afraid of dying during intercourse. Exact figures are difficult to obtain, especially since all kinds of horror stories are told. More often than not, such deaths occur in extra-marital affairs. The findings of the relatively few studies on this topic show that death rarely occurs during intercourse. A Japanese study of 5,559 cases of sudden death showed that 34 occurred during sexual activity and that of these 34 patients, 18 had coronary heart disease. Of these 18 sudden deaths, 80% occurred during extra-marital affairs, and 50% occurred in a hotel. What conclusion can we draw from these statistics?

Surrounding circumstances

In our opinion, the risk of a re-infarction during intercourse is not great. The sex act itself poses a lesser risk than accompanying circumstances. These may include excessive food and alcohol intake, and nicotine abuse, as well as guilt, fear of being discovered, and being in strange surroundings with a different partner to whom one's potency must be proven. We advise our patients to eliminate the uncomfortable circumstances as much as possible if the sexual activities cannot be resumed in a comfortable marital situation. Excesses of drinking and eating should be avoided, the location should be secure, and the time should be chosen carefully, not after a heavy meal and in the morning rather than in the evening. The encounter should be based on tenderness, fun, and enjoyment.

Bring tenderness into play

The delicate subject of extra-marital affairs after a heart attack should also be discussed with the physician. He should not neglect this topic since it is important for many patients. Already in 1948, the Kinsey Report showed that in the 1930's and 1940's half of the married men and 25% of married women had extra-marital

116

affairs.

Heart attack patients who are single, widowed, divorced, old or homosexual, also rarely discuss sexuality with their physician. We urge these patients to raise the topic, especially since physicians are sometimes grateful when a patient initiates the conversation. Often such conversations provoke the physician to consider his own attitude toward sexuality. Must sex always have reproduction as its goal? How should a physician who is happily married counsel a patient who has extra-marital affairs? Does a younger physician believe that older patients are no longer interested in sex?

It is more difficult to give sexual counsel to heart attack patients who recover very slowly than it is to counsel those who can attain 75 watts or more on a bicycle ergometer and easily readjust to daily life again. In such cases we suggest that the patient gradually resume sexual activity. For some patients, masturbation may be the answer. Studies have shown that masturbation involves less exertion, and that in this way men can discover whether they are capable of erection and women can discover whether orgasm is possible.

The advising physician often encounters religious opposition and preconceived notions about normal sexuality. Older women in particular fear perversity and are very inhibited. Even though it is generally known that masturbation causes no physical or emotional harm, many who masturbate feel guilty, do not discuss it with their partner, and do not help the partner masturbate.

Libido and potency are also influenced by the patient's general depression and loss of self-confidence in the weeks and months following the heart attack. The patient fears failure, but then makes no attempt to succeed. Men in particular can develop such an anxiety about impotence that they are in fact impotent during the decisive moment. Problems with potency develop in 90% of the cases as a result of both the pressure to perform and the fear of impotence. Many men make the mistake of concentrating on the erection rather than the tenderness they give and the pleasure they hope for.

If sex is viewed as an accomplishment rather than as a mutual experience, then the fear of failure will ruin the joy of tenderness, touching, embracing, stroking, and caressing. In our opinion the discussions with patients and spouses should concentrate not only on technique (for example, the more suitable side-to-side position),

Discuss this with your physician

Masturbation is more than substitute

Fear of failure can be reduced

117

but also on their wishes and apprehensions. The spouse must be included in the conversation because the attitude of the partners toward each other and to sex will play an important role. Few problems with potency result when sexuality is viewed positively by both partners, if both enjoy the physical contact, and if their fears are allayed.

The coronary patient as a spoiled child

To achieve a happy sexual relationship, the coronary patient should not act like a spoiled child, constantly demanding attention from his spouse. The origin of such a role can often be found in the situation prior to the heart attack and the blame should often be shared by the patient, spouse and physician. On the other hand, the wife may treat the patient like a substitute child because the heart attack often occurs at a time when the children have left the house. The physician sometimes encourages this mothering role of the wife when he makes her responsible for the patient's diet, normal weight, non-smoking, daily exercise, protection, and taking of medication. As a result, the wife of a patient who was previously the active, domineering sexual partner may no longer be content with her passive sexual role when she must take care of him all day long.

The sexual relationship may also be altered when the wife takes over the patient's financial business, and especially when the patient had equated manhood with such duties. Many men feel guilty when they are no longer able to provide for the family. They have mixed feelings about the changing role of the wife and feel uneasy when the wife makes independent decisions. The wife may have guilt feelings because she pays more attention to the husband than to the children or because she is irritable when she cannot fulfill expectations. She may also become irritable either when she shows her fears, or when she must conceal them in order not to burden others.

Sexual and personal life-fulfillment

Despite all these problems and uncertainties, many patients are able to make the heart attack the beginning of an especially good relationship. Such a relationship is possible if all fears are discussed openly either with or without the physician's presence.

118

In fact, relations with spouse and children may become more profound and intense after the heart attack. As far as sex is concerned, the patient may recognize how monotonous contact had become, and may then learn to take more time for sex and to cultivate new tenderness in caressing. The male patient may then reflect on his role and learn to establish greater equality between the partners. As a result, many heart attack patients discover a better life-style in which sexuality and greater potency play an important role.

Remember what is important in life

Although sex may currently be over-emphasized, it does play a fundamental role in human existence. For more people, whether they are young or old, healthy or sick, sexuality is part of personal life-fulfillment and is a means of achieving happiness with another person. The physician should discuss this topic with the patient because it requires great care and thought even for healthy persons.

Work and Social Life

The following statement is made on the basis of long experience in rehabilitation:

Old place of work or new job?

Both hourly wage-earners and those who are self-employed should continue their previous work. For those who have just sustained a heart attack it is best to return to their old place of work or at least to their previous employer.

However, in many cases a worker's ability is assessed according to psychological rather than physiological criteria. As a result, it is wrong to give general advice based solely on objective physical ability as estimated, for instance, by ergometry. As an example of the necessity to judge each case individually, we cite the case of a young man who is physically fit but must be dismissed as a result of a neurosis, whereas another man with severe coronary heart disease is able to work satisfactorily for ten hours a day. A

Problems for self-employment

self-employed person may lose what he has carefully built up over the years if he is away from his work for a long period of time and if he is not adequately covered by insurance. In most cases the patient can return to work within three to six months after the heart attack if he had not experienced complications within four to six weeks following the attack.

119

In the Hoehenried long-term study of 1,000 patients 80% of blue-collar and 90% of white collar workers were able to resume their work. If conflicts and situations of psychosocial stress develop, the patient should attempt to change his working conditions. For example, his responsibilities could be reduced or he could take up other duties. In our opinion it is important that the physician speak with both the employer and co-workers in order to determine what would be best for the patient. Frequently social responsibilities are involved in holding a particular job, but the patient must then decide which social functions or honorary positions are important. He should discuss this subject with his spouse, friends, and physician.

Conflicts at work

Leisure Time and Vacation

When can I drive again?

Driving your own car

This question is frequently posed by those patients who are dependent on a car for transportation to work or who live in areas where public transportation is not available.

● We let our patients drive a private car three months after a heart attack without complications.

The patient's personal attitude toward driving, traffic, and speed is more important than the amount of time that has elapsed since the heart attack. How might he react in a difficult situation? Much depends on whether the patient enjoys driving or becomes nervous, causing his pulse and blood pressure to rise. Heavy city traffic does not disturb a good driver who is relaxed. Of course, there are certain unhealthy accompanying factors such as exhaust fumes, noise, and frustration resulting from traffic jams and inconsiderate drivers.

If the patient takes anticoagulants, he should always carry information on his medication, prothrombin values and blood group with him.

Restrictions for professional drivers

These suggestions are self-evident for those who drive private vehicles. Much stricter regulations apply to those who drive to earn their living.

Am I allowed to fly?

If no complications arise, then patients may fly six to eight weeks

120

after the heart attack. Recommendations vary from one country to another. In modern, pressurized airplanes, a flight of one to three hours may be allowed after three weeks following the attack. In general, flights are tolerated better than the patient assumes. If flights posed any special dangers, then certainly this news would be well-known among patients. However, international flights should be chosen with greater care because tolerance for longer travel is lower after a heart attack. Great time differences and a hot, humid climate may pose particular problems. If a patient notices that he feels progressively worse after each flight (if he develops chest pains and they become increasingly severe), then he should contact his physician immediately. Since such pain is a warning signal, a thorough examination should be made.

Be careful with international flights

When can I participate in sports again?

This question must be answered individually by a physician experienced in sports. The answer depends not only on the type of sport you practice (football, tennis, golf, skiing, or bowling), but also on your recovery from the heart attack, such as whether there are irregularities of the cardiac rhythm or other complications and how well you perform on the bicycle ergometer test. If everything goes well with your recovery, then you can probably take up your favorite sports again a year after the heart attack. You should not, however, engage in competitive sports, but play for fun.

No competitive sports

When can I participate in parties and dances again?

Parties and informal gatherings are a good way for you to renew your social contacts and enjoy life. Such social activities can be harmful only if you lose your self-control and eat or drink too much, or smoke cigarettes. Dancing is in fact an ideal form of controlled exercise. We give our patients the opportunity to dance every day for relaxation and have not experienced any adverse effects. We suggest that patients who tend to develop angina pectoris take nitrates as a preventive measure before dancing.

Dancing relaxes

Can I watch TV again?

In our experience, complications are more likely to develop when the patient watches exciting football games or crime stories than when he dances. Each patient should judge for himself whether certain television shows are potentially harmful because he is overly excitable.

Too much excitement

121

Where and how should I spend my vacation?

Patients who have either sustained a heart attack or are threatened by one, should choose a moderate climate and altitudes below 5,000 feet. For many years, heart attack patients were advised not to go higher than 3,300 feet, but our experience has shown that this height can be ideal for the patient since he can thus escape the fog during winter and the hot humidity during summer. Those patients who ski well and have recovered without complications may generally participate in ski and glacier tours a year after the heart attack.

A moderate climate is preferable

Sometimes restful vacations are distinguished from those characterized by a great deal of activity, but, of course, the vacation of a heart attack patient should contain both elements. The patient must carefully balance physical activity and relaxation by getting a good night's rest and a nap in the afternoon. If the patient has difficulty falling asleep in a different location, he should take a mild sleeping pill for the first few days.

Appendix

Herbs for Salt-Free, Low-Salt Diets

(All of the material included in this appendix is taken, with the kind permission of the publishers, from **Herbs—Nature's Own Seasonings,** *copyright © 1978, by the Herb Society of Hilton Head Island. For further information, write to The Herb Society, P.O. Box 5765, Hilton Head Island, SC 29928.)*

Try these favorites for starters

Basil—a spicy, clove-like taste and scent. Use it with zucchini and in tomato dishes, soups, stews. Toss liberally into spaghetti and salads.

Bay—one leaf or a pinch, fresh or dried, improves nearly all savory dishes—vegetable soups, stews, pot roasts . . .

Burnet—cucumber-flavored. Slip it in wherever you want a delicate cucumbery taste—in salads, of course; iced drinks, herb spreads.

Chervil—parsley-like with its own intriguing flavor. A fine addition to soups, stews and salads. A delicate herb, useful in blends.

Chives (garlic and regular)—Ever useful and more subtle than their onion cousins. Keep on hand at all times—fresh or frozen. Garlic chives have special importance: for those who cannot digest garlic, here's a fine substitute.

Coriander—use the seeds, crushed, for a delightful addition to baked fruits, peas, stews.

Dill—goes with almost everything, both leaves and seeds. Superb with fish. Chop over tomatoes, cucumbers and yogurt. Try on lamb chops, in cottage cheese.

123

Fennel—a licoricey hint that gives a lift to salads, soups and particularly fish dishes. Seeds are good in omelets, sauerkraut, salad dressings. An alter-ego for dill.

Marjoram—sweet, tangy taste is a natural for eggplant, summer squash, zucchini, pastas. Sprinkle over veal chops and chicken. Flavors almost all but sweet dishes. A good blending herb.

Mint—comes in a variety of flavors with delicious aroma. Snip into salads, fresh fruits, peas, meatballs. Add to teas.

Oregano—the spicy "pizza" herb, an Italian and Spanish standby. It asserts itself in no uncertain terms. Great in meat dishes, with mushrooms, broccoli, zucchini.

Parsley—not just a garnish. It's a delicious ingredient of soups, sauces, herb spreads, cottage cheese. Team with chopped garlic for French long-cook dishes. High in Vitamin C. Can be a salad in itself.

Rosemary—a strong, distinctive taste and aroma. Goes with beef, lamb, chicken, turkey. Boil with old potatoes; toss with peas and cauliflower and minestrone-type soups. Lay a sprig on spinach when you cook it.

Sage—the pungent staple of stuffings, roasted meats. Throw a big leaf in when you're cooking peas. Sprinkle on brussels sprouts. Can be used inside a roasting chicken.

Savory—Summer and winter-types (the latter is a bit stronger). Try with beans and cabbage, in scrambled eggs, fish chowders and sauces.

Tarragon—lends authority to salad dressings, vinegars, herb spreads, all fish and shellfish, baked or broiled. Sprinkle lightly over poultry before roasting. Blends well with chervil and chives. If you grow this, be sure the variety is French—fragrant and tasty—not Russian which is neither.

Thyme—the chef's meat and poultry secret. It's all-around, aromatic, a nice surprise with onions and eggplant. Lemon thyme, a variety you must grow yourself (it does not come packaged), is an excellent blending herb—delicious on fish, along with marjoram.

Other seasonings to bring out food flavors

Ginger Root—a real mystery ingredient. Its special spicy flavor does wonders for almost anything. Sold in many supermarkets now. Keep refrigerated, frozen or immersed in sherry wine; then grate off a bit as you need it for meats (superb on steak), fish, turkey, vegetables, fruit desserts. Use in combination with all herbs to heighten a food's taste. Ground ginger can be substituted, but has less punch.

Curry—a dash of this multi-spice blend is one secret that brings many foods to life. Use it in soups, cottage cheese, salad dressings, meat marinades, eggs, vegetable dishes. It doesn't shine through—just gives character.

Dry Mustard—adds snap to vegetables, meat marinades, salad dressings, cream sauces for eggs and poultry. Rub some over lamb chops, ham, and pork roasts.

Sesame Seeds (Benne to Southerners)—Toast these in a slow oven before using. This brings out the nutlike flavor. Then pop into fish and chicken dishes, mixtures of vegetables. Sprinkle on salads.

Lime—give lemons a rest and use lime instead. Adds a distinctive delicious twist. Consider this as a discovery.

Nutmeg—a "must" in Greek and Middle Eastern cooking. A real dividend in meatballs, cheese sauces, fruit salad, spinach and other vegetables.

Pepper—of course! You'll get the best from fresh peppercorns. Crush them to release the good oils.

The Zests—lemon and orange, marvelous to have on hand when you need grated peel and/or juice. An addition to herbal teas.

Lemon Verbena—an excellent herb for bringing a hint of lemon to any recipe.

Mint Essence—a handy way to add mint to iced tea, hot tea, carrots, peas, meats, fresh fruits. Steep a handful of fresh mint leaves in a cup of boiling water. Cool, strain and bottle. Store in refrigerator for use.

Shallots—onion relatives with their own special touch. Store in a hanging mesh bag. If they begin to sprout, plant in dirt until you are ready to use them. If shallots are not available, rub garden green onion with cut clove of garlic as a substitute.

Eight good spices to experiment with: allspice, cinnamon, cloves and **mace**—all fragrant and spicy-sweet; **paprika-**many varieties, use for color and pungency; **cayenne**—a pinch packs a punch; **saffron**—important to bouillabaisse, many French, Spanish and Italian dishes; **turmeric**—saffron-like, a good substitute.

Tips from the Experts

- Keep a light hand on herbs in the beginning. It's best to start out mildly, then develop daring.
- Herbs, after drying, are best stored in airtight containers, in a dry place, away from heat and sunlight.
- When you use dried herbs instead of fresh, cut the quantity in half.
- One-half teaspoon of dried herbs will season one pint of sauce, one pint of soup or one pound of meat. This is a conservative usage; as you experiment, you may want more.
- Make crushing herbs easy by equipping yourself with a mortar and pestle or a handy little hand-turned grinder designed specifically for herbs.
- To revive the flavor of long-stored herbs, soak for 10 minutes in one teaspoon of lemon juice.
- Poaching a fish? Try a sprig of fennel in the stock, along with lemon thyme or marjoram.
- When a recipe calls for unavailable shallots, substitute a green onion rubbed with the cut side of a clove of garlic. The effect is close.
- At what point do you add herbs to a dish? If it's a long, slow cooker, such as soup, add them later for maximum effect. If it's uncooked or cold, the sooner, the better.
- A bay leaf slipped into opened containers of flour, rice and other staples will keep the bugs out.
- Sprinkle a tablespoon of mint leaves (chopped) on top of a mixed vegetable or fruit salad.
- Depend on herb vinegars. A dash gives unexpected taste to vegetables, salad dressings, meat marinades. And they come (or you can make them) based on wine or non-wine, flavored with such herbs as basil, mint, burnet, tarragon, plus shallots, garlic and spices.
- If you use herbs on a meat dish, try them in another form on the vegetables, herb vinegar, for example, or one of the herb spreads (margarine with a blend of herbs).
- Serve fresh or frozen produce whenever possible. The processing of food often adds salt and calories and subtracts nutrition. If canned food must be used, you can eliminate excess salt and sugar by rinsing with water.

Index